To Turn You On

39 Sex Fantasies For Women

BY J. APHRODITE

BARRICADE
BOOKS

Published by Barricade Books Inc.
2037 Lemoine Avenue
Fort Lee, New Jersey 07024

www.barricadebooks.com

Library of Congress Cataloging-in-Publication Data

Aphrodite, J.
  To turn you on : 39 sex fantasies for women / J. Aphrodite.
    pages cm
  ISBN 978-1-56980-580-0
  1. Erotic stories, American. I. Title.
  PS3551.P35T6 2015
  813'.54--dc23
                                                         2015004769

10 9 8 7 6 5 4 3 2 1
Manufactured in the United States of America

*To the women of the world . . . and
especially to those who know that a primary
goal in life is to find as much
enjoyment as possible.*

The ultimate value of a book of this sort is in its practical application. This volume was tested in manuscript form among friends and strangers and I want to express my warm gratitude to Peggy, Marilyn, Sherri, Marie-Claude, Jackie, Joy, Alby, Becky, Joan, Pat and Gerda, among others, for sharing with me some of their most intimate daydreams.

I particularly want to express my thanks to my publisher for encouraging me to continue this bold project in the face of loss of confidence and to Sandra Lee Stuart, my editor, for setting me straight when I had lost my direction.

J.A.

TABLE OF CONTENTS

Why this book?

IS THERE A woman alive who would deny, even to herself, that she has ever had a sexual daydream? There was a time when women would be reluctant to express their sexuality. But all has changed. With the publication of books like "Fifty Shades of Grey," and others, women are encouraged to enjoy their fantasies. And now, with "TO TURN YOU ON" I hope I will have added pleasure to their lives.

For many years, like other young women, I felt it was my function to serve my partner. My sexual satisfaction was secondary.

I wasn't often satisfied. But I thought that was how things had to be. But soon, books began to appear talking about women and their fantasies. Many were all thickly coated with pretension. They skirted the real world of sexual fantasy. And they failed to stimulate me. What you will find in this book is a collection of fantasies designed to turn you on.

Not all of the fantasies in this book are mine. I talked with women I knew and virtually all admitted they had sex fantasies that often helped them to achieve more pleasure with their partners. Some of the fantasies in this book are those shared by those women.

What I also learned is that a fantasy is a fantasy only when it lives in the imagination. We do not want most of our fantasies to come true. There is no claim that all of them are universal. Or that the collection touches all bases. This is an assortment. It is my assortment. There should be something here for everyone.

If these set you off on your own sexual daydreams, either when you are with your favorite man or woman, or when you are alone — if they further the emergence of your sexual assertiveness—if they turn *you* on—then I have succeeded in doing what I have set out to do. Enjoy.

J.A.

How to Read This Book

A COLLECTION OF SEX fantasies is not the sort of book to curl up with in your armchair and read from cover to cover in one evening. Rather, it should be ingested only after anticipation and planning. The fantasies should also be read slowly—no more than two or three at a sitting.

Don't take this book with you to read while waiting your turn at the dentist, or during coffee break at the office, or while hanging on to a subway strap during rush hour. It will all go to waste.

These fantasies are simple to read and easy to understand. Yet an incredible amount of research and care went in to making them that way. What I'd like you to do is to set aside a half hour when you have time all to yourself. Open to the table of contents and let a title or two catch your fancy.

Then, curl up in that chair—or better yet—lie on the sofa or between the sheets in your bed and read slowly. Afterwards, close the book and close your eyes. Relive the fantasy in your imagination and your imagination will add personal variations. Let your imagination run free and it will show you the way to whatever pleasure follows.

Remember—my hope is that these fantasies will give you hours of pleasure . . . nothing more, and nothing less . . .

First Experience

YOU WERE FOURTEEN. Fourteen and four months (to be exact)! You don't remember when you first became aware of the noises coming from the bedroom across the hall, but it must have easily been a year ago. You tiptoed to the door of your parents' room and at first only listened. Both your father and mother were making the same sounds you'd heard so often. Your father was breathing very heavily and once in a while, he'd grunt. And your mother was saying "Ohhhhhhh" over and over.

For many weeks it became a nightly preoccupation. Your imagination was vivid and you could just see them in all kinds of sexual positions. Wow! You hadn't realized your churchgoing mother would do all those sexy things that raced through your mind!

After listening, you'd tiptoe back to bed and under the covers massage your vagina with one hand while pulling gently at your budding nipples with the other.

Then one night there was a surprise. That night your parents left the bedside lamp on. You saw light coming from beneath the door and at first were almost afraid to approach it. But you were drawn to it like a moth to a flame. You looked through the keyhole. It was a sight you would never forget. Your mother was on her back with her legs all the way up in the air, leaning them against your father's shoulders. Your father was between her legs moving in and out against her. Suddenly—uncontrollably—you sneezed!

"What was that?" you heard your mother say.

You were too frozen to move, but you stared as your father pulled out of your mother and you glimpsed his penis swinging in the air with white liquid at the end of it. He came toward the door and you scampered back to your room.

"Nothing there," you heard him say above the pounding of your heart, as he swung the door open and shut again.

You never dared venture to the door again. But you would lie awake at night caressing yourself and wondering what it would feel like to have someone do those things to you.

It was on your very first date when you would begin to find out.

Rudy, an eighteen year old who played on the basketball team, asked you to a dance. The dance was poorly attended and he wanted to know if you'd like to leave and go to see a movie. You told him sure.

You made conversation all the while to cover your self-consciousness. In the theater, you sat on the side, quite apart from other people.

For a long time you just watched the movie, and then you realized that you were so conscious of Rudy being next to you that you hadn't even been aware of the actor smiling out at you from the screen.

After a while, awkwardly, Rudy put his arm on the seat in back of you. You froze. Then, imperceptibly, you leaned back. You sensed his hand moving closer to your shoulder and then it was against your bare skin. Meanwhile, he stared straight at the screen as if he wasn't aware of what his left arm was doing.

The arm pulled you close to him and you moved without resistance. When he turned and looked at you, chills went all over you. He leaned down and kissed you. You wanted him to kiss you again. You knew at that moment that you loved him.

But he moved back and seemed to be watching the movie again. Soon, with your head resting on his shoulder, you felt his fingers move closer to the center of your blouse and slowly ease under it until he had lifted up your light bra and had his hand on your breast. You were absolutely motionless. Then his other hand was on your left breast. He was pulling gently at the nipple and letting his finger go up and down over it. His hand slid over to the other breast and began to do the same things. You heard your own breathing. You placed your hand over his and pressed it tighter against your breast. Then you felt his other hand on your thigh—as if it had just dropped there accidentally—without purpose.

Soon you felt the hand moving under your skirt. Involuntarily, your legs spread as his fingers reached the crotch of your panties. The fingers played on the outside and you sank lower into the chair. Then a stray finger slipped underneath and began caressing your pubic hair, which was so soft and downy. The rest of the fingers joined in and you had to control yourself as his hand reached between your legs, stretching the panties high while he slowly moved up and down on your mound. Your eyes closed. There was a flow of wet juices which you didn't quite understand, but it all felt so good . . . and you seemed to just float away. . . .

Suddenly you became aware that the film was ending. Rudy withdrew his hands as the lights went on. He leaned over and kissed you again and you tried to press your right breast against him.

Then, as if nothing at all had happened, he said, "Did you like the movie?"

"Oh yes," you murmured.

"Let's go to another one soon, okay?"

"Yes," you said softly, "*very* soon."

2

Your Best Friend's Husband

YOU WERE ANGRY with yourself for being so helpless since the divorce. You never realized how many things Tim had taken care of; things which you didn't have the foggiest notion how to handle. Now the sink was stuffed up and the superintendent had the day off. You sat there looking at the mess. Tears of frustration were beginning to form in the corners of your eyes.

Then you remembered what Jill had said shortly after the divorce: If you had any problems, or needed anything, she or Don would be happy to help out. Even though you knew she meant it, you were always reluctant to ask for anything. You were worried that one day if you really needed something, you would have worn out your welcome. But the horrid mess kept staring back at you, so hesitantly you picked up the phone.

"Oh sure, as soon as Don is finished with dinner, I'll ask him to go on up," Jill replied, obviously happy to help a friend.

The two of you lived only three floors apart in this apartment building, and you'd gotten to be very good friends over the years. She and Don had been helpful during the separation and were eager to show you that they were still your friends, even though you were now without a husband. You appreciated this, since it was a tough adjustment for you. At the age of forty-three you probably should have felt more self-confidence, but being left by Tim for a younger woman didn't help your self-image.

Within fifteen minutes Don was standing at your door with

a plunger in his hand and a friendly smile on his face. As he entered, you suddenly were aware of how sloppy you looked. You'd fallen into the habit of putting on that old bathrobe as soon as you came home. Being alone most evenings, you didn't pay much attention to "dressing." (You made a mental note to change that attitude.. . .) You felt awkward, but you dismissed it as you led Don to the sink.

"I'll fix that in a hurry," he said, and you sat down in the kitchen to watch and kibbitz.

As he worked, he chatted. He took a couple of quick peeks at your bare legs, but only in a very casual way.

"Say, Jill has been asking you to dinner for weeks, but you never say yes. How about it? Don't keep isolating yourself."

"I guess you're right," you replied. "I *have* been staying in too much. I'll say yes next time."

In short order the sink was unstuffed and the mess disappeared down the drain. Don asked if you had any rags to clean up with.

You kept the box of rags on top of one of the shelves in the storage room off the kitchen. As you climbed up on the step stool to reach it, you felt a hand underneath your robe. You screamed as you spun around, totally caught off guard. You found yourself staring into Don's faintly amused eyes.

"Hey, cut it out. That's not funny."

"I didn't mean to be funny," he answered coolly. "I only wanted to see if your legs felt as smooth as they look."

"Well, I don't appreciate that," you stammered and tried to climb down, but Don was there in front of you, not moving.

"In fact," he continued, "I think I'm going to fuck you."

You had no reply to this one. He looked like he wasn't kidding, but you tried to joke him out of it, "Oh, come on Don, Jill is my best friend—you're my good friend, wouldn't that be silly?"

But he stood his ground.

The next move was Don swiftly untying your robe and revealing your nude body.

You grappled with him, trying to close the robe, but he took both your wrists in one hand and held them in a painfully tight grip. You protested—told him he was hurting you, and begged him to let go. He answered that he would, but only if you didn't fight him.

"I can't . . . please don't do this," you pleaded. And then you were sobbing like a child. All the frustration you felt for being alone so often and so helpless, and now *this* just overwhelmed you. Don didn't seem to care. He pulled you down from the stool, still holding your wrists, and led you into your bedroom.

After he threw you onto the bed and pulled off your robe, he started to undress himself. His grip loosened slightly, enabling you to wrench yourself free and to run for the door. You thought that if you could get out, you'd go for help. But he was quicker than you, and once again you were back on the bed. He slapped you across the face for having tried to run and you sobbed as your face grew red from the blow. Now he used his belt to tie your hands together. He held onto the strap, controlling your hands.

He quickly lowered his pants. He was already hard and you stared at him with fear and hatred.

Once more you pleaded for him to stop, but he said nothing. He pushed you down and climbed onto the bed. The tears were coming without stopping now. In a sudden movement he pushed his penis into your mouth until you choked on it. With one hand he held onto the strap while the other hand had you by the back of the head. He pushed himself in and out of your mouth roughly, each time causing you to choke and gag. You looked up to see his eyes fixed on you, obviously getting very excited by the sight of his penis raping your mouth.

When it seemed that he was about to come, he stopped and moved away. He fastened the strap to the headboard so that your hands were now trussed above your head. He forced your legs up over his shoulders as he positioned himself between them.

How you hated him! You turned your face away and shut your eyes tightly so you wouldn't have to look at him. As he entered you, his penis penetrated so deeply it felt as if it would reach your stomach. He withdrew it almost to its tip and then quickly thrust it into you again. He kept on, each time withdrawing it slowly, so slowly, and then rushing back into you. You heard him breathing harder and harder.

He reached for your nipples and began to pinch and pull them. In spite of yourself they responded. You wanted to die of shame. After fucking you and pinching your nipples for a long time, he moved his one free hand down. It traced a line from between your breasts and past your navel to your pubic hair. It rested there a moment before he began to manipulate your clitoris. Just as your nipples had responded, it also began tingling. God! It had been so long since any man had touched you.

He felt the hard tip of your clit and all at once his fucking became slower but with a decidedly steady rhythm. He kept rubbing and pulling at your clit until you felt your body imitating his. Soon it was no longer only his breathing you heard, but your own as well.

You melted now and forgot about how it all began. You weren't sure how long he continued, but it seemed to be only a moment before you were about to arrive. You shuddered and moaned as your orgasm was triggered. He was carried along with it and came at once, filling you with his semen.

A few minutes later he was dressing, and you, untied, were lying limp on the bed.

He smiled but said nothing. You both knew neither of you

would say anything about the incident to Jill. It would be his word against yours, and he would convince her that you had enticed him.

But you also knew that you would always be able to call on Don if you needed anything fixed.

3

Visit To The Gynecologist

YOUR LAST VISIT to Doctor Gordon took place more than a year ago. Now it was time for another routine checkup by the gynecologist. Much had happened in the last year—you had lost weight, gained confidence in yourself, and looked quite different. Your hair was longer, and you had tinted it to a shade of red that made heads turn when you walked down the street. Your makeup was more professional, too, and your eyes were particularly outstanding—the soft black liner you used made their very light blue color even more noticeable. Your style of dressing had become more sensuous; you now favored clingy fabrics and close-fitting slacks. You wondered if Doctor Gordon would notice the change in you. He was very handsome, you'd always thought—but very professional.

As you sat in the waiting room, you smiled to yourself, remembering the schoolgirl crush you had always had on him. You figured it happened to almost every woman—falling in love with her gynecologist—but your feeling hadn't dissipated. Here it was, a full year since you'd last visited him, and you felt your heart beating faster just wondering if he still looked the same.

Talk about greying at the temples and all that! He had a year-round tan which he maintained by skiing in the winter and sailing in the summer. He was clean shaven and always looked spotless, with blue eyes that added to his virile image. The short-sleeved shirts he wore showed off his strong arms to their best advantage.

The nurse interrupted your daydreams by calling out your name. She led you into one of the examining rooms where you were to remove all your clothing. You started to disrobe but hadn't quite finished when the door opened and Doctor Gordon walked in. There you were, in your bra, with one foot in and one foot out of your bikini panties when you froze.

"Sorry," he said, "I thought you were ready for me."

"Uh, uh, that's okay," you muttered and hurried along.

Finishing quickly, you stood nude for a moment and thought you caught him glance at you. You went up to the examining table and looked for the robe that was usually there, but couldn't find it.

"Oh, I think we can dispense with that," he said and offered you a hand in getting up onto the table.

"You seem to have reduced your weight since I last examined you," he remarked.

"Yes," you said and silently cursed the blush that swept over you.

"No need to be embarrassed," he said. "You look very well."

"Thank you" was all you could think to say.

"Now move down to the end of the table and put your feet here," he said. He gently helped you move your hips to the edge as you got into the position for the examination.

He began to professionally knead and prod your breasts. As he finished, you could have sworn you felt his hand brush past your nipples. But surely you must have imagined it. . . .

Then he moved down to the end of the table. He was very gentle and thorough and asked several routine questions. Then his questions took a different turn.

"How are your sexual responses?" he asked.

Although you were startled, he was, after all, your doctor, and you assumed he wanted to know for some professional reason.

"Well, fine, I guess."

"Let's see," he said and then his finger was deep inside you—deeper than you thought was possible. He began to manipulate your insides and asked, "Does this feel good?" The sensation from his fingering made you feel fantastic and helpless at the same time. It started to grow and grow but you didn't know what to do about it. You didn't want to be lying there on his table with an orgasm about to erupt.

"Relax," he said, his voice very soft now. "Do you feel like you're going to have an orgasm?"

"Well—yes," you sputtered.

"Fine, fine," he said, "just see if you can relax and let it happen."

"I don't think I can," you replied.

"Well, try. I'll help you."

So you closed your eyes and pretended that you were not in a doctor's office. And again the warm tingling sensation began. His finger was working in you relentlessly.

His body was pressing on you ever so slightly as he leaned against the table.

"Let it happen," he kept saying, "let yourself come. . . ."

And then—you did. An orgasm rushed over your body, and you shivered with the suddenness of it. But he didn't stop. He kept moving his finger and urging you to try once more.

"See if you can do it again," he said and his voice was even more hushed. "I'll try something different now."

That same tantalizing finger continued to excite you, but now his other hand moved against your clitoris, gently at first, just brushing past it back and forth. The rhythm of both hands was hypnotizing—the back and forth pulsation of one while the other teased your clitoris. And then there was something wet and soft at your clit, and you realized that it was his mouth and he was licking you. You didn't know whether to jump off the table or to protest or what. So you kept your eyes closed and let him go on.

His tongue on the outside and his finger inside, were taking you higher and higher. You felt the licking increase in intensity—your clitoris hardened, your body tensed, and you knew you were about to come again. You were moving to meet his tongue and his finger, and you heard soft purring sounds escape from deep within you. Suddenly you were into another marvelous orgasm which went on forever because he wouldn't stop his licking and fingering. You kept coming until you couldn't bear any more.

Then he gently pulled out his finger and stopped with his mouth. You opened your eyes and saw his face was very flushed. But his voice was professional and crisp as he said, "Well, I think your responses are fine, but you should really come in to see me about once a month so I can make sure everything continues this way."

And he turned and left the room, leaving you to dress.

4

The Masseuse

WHAT A TIRING day at the office! How you've looked forward to unwinding at your health club. Even as you ride the hot, uncomfortable subway, your mind is on the shower you'll soon take, followed by a sauna where you'll just lie for a while, as all the weariness ebbs from your body. Today you're going to treat yourself to a massage—something you save for those special occasions, when you really need a pick-me-up.

At last you're at the club. You book a massage, giving yourself an hour to get ready at a relaxed pace. There's a new masseuse, Ingrid, a German girl. Well that's fine, as long as she gives you a good, firm working over.

You shower and rest in the sauna and feel the-weariness leave your body. Lying there alone in the dry heat, you mentally take stock of yourself. Not bad, you think; medium breasts which are still quite firm with nipples that stand up at the slightest erotic thought, let alone touch. Flat stomach with hipbones that protrude in a rather sexy way. Your pubic hair is very thick—something that used to embarrass you until you discovered how many men were turned on by it. You were lucky with your legs—even though you were close to forty, they were your pride and joy. Long and slim with no ugly veins. You were just drifting off to sleep when you hear your name being called. Massage time . . .

Almost reluctantly you shower again, afterwards wrapping yourself in a large terry cloth towel. Ingrid smiles shyly at you as if in introduction. You smile too and she somehow

indicates that she speaks very little English. She leads you to
a private cubicle and helps you up onto the table. She draws
the curtains and you let your eyes close in anticipation of the
delicious feeling you will receive as soon as Ingrid begins to
manipulate your flesh.

You're face down. Ingrid removes the towel. You wait for the
sheet that normally is draped over the parts of your body not
being massaged, but it never arrives. Well, you say to yourself,
I guess this is the German way. There is a long pause and you
get a tiny uneasy feeling — as if your body were being carefully
scrutinized. But soon Ingrid's strong hands are working on
your shoulders and you cast out this silly notion.

She's quite good at her job, and you relax as she works over
your neck and arms and back. It's delightful. Then you feel
her hands on your buttocks. They move gently at first and
then more firmly. You wonder if she isn't spending too much
time on them, but you dismiss this thought and just enjoy it.
Every once in a while you feel her fingers just brush lightly
between your cheeks and a tingle runs through you and then
quickly vanishes. Now Ingrid is working on your legs. She
works upward, starting with your toes, then instep, ankles,
calves, and knees. She takes the tension out of your thighs
with her strong hands. Then she does something you've never
experienced in a massage — she places her hands on the insides
of your thighs, rubbing first down and then up — over and
over. You feel the tips of her fingers brushing your pubic hair.

Before you can protest, Ingrid is indicating that you should
turn on your back. As you do, you open your eyes slightly and
it seems to you that Ingrid's face is somewhat flushed. Probably from exhaustion, you think, as you shut your eyes again.

She begins with your face and works quickly down to your
neck and shoulders. Smoothing your shoulders and arms,
she moves expertly and soon is massaging the sensitive skin
alongside the outer part of your breasts. She takes some more

of the cream she has been using and begins to make circles around your breasts with both her hands. You feel your nipples respond. You know how easily they do, but this once you wish they wouldn't stand out so far and hard.

You take a peek at Ingrid who is very obviously and lustfully looking at your body. Your instinct is to jump off the massage table and run, but instead you decide to allow her to finish. If you can get through this without her knowing that you see how turned on she is, you'll just never come back to her table. Finally, Ingrid moves her hands away from your breasts and continues downward. You are relieved but you have to admit that it felt good. You're quite shaken at this discovery.

Before it can worry you more, you feel her working on your legs again, this time from the top—and again her hands are on the insides of your thighs, massaging firmly, and again her fingertips are brushing against your pubic hair. All at once you hear a slight moan escape your lips. You know she must have heard this, too, and again you want to run. But you just lie there mastered by her strong, insistent hands. Again you open your eyes slightly and catch a tiny smile crossing Ingrid's lips. She knows you're enjoying it.

For just a moment your eyes meet and then she moves her probing, ceaseless hands with even more vigor. Her fingers are brushing past your pubic hair and reaching lightly for your clitoris. It tautens immediately. You close your eyes, afraid to do anything. You feel your vagina moisten. Her fingers slip easily over your clitoris and into you. You sigh softly, and Ingrid's strokes become steady and hypnotically exciting.

She spreads your legs by placing herself between them, making you totally vulnerable to her. You feel those fingers in and out and then you almost leap from the table as her tongue flicks over the tip of your clitoris. She licks you again and your body arches. She relaxes then into a rhythm that is completely new to you. Her tongue touches every part of your vagina—the clitoris, the outer lips, the inner lips, and then darts in and out of the opening. Over and over again she works away at you as you drift into a trance. Then she reaches up with her hands and begins to rub your breasts, all the while licking you. She sucks your juices and wets you again and again with her tongue. You feel yourself getting closer and closer to the climactic summit when she begins tongue-teasing you—slowing up until she makes you plead with your body for her to continue. You move your wet bush closer to her face and she responds, moving her tongue, harder and faster as she licks at all the right spots—her hands still moving in circles on your breasts. You feel yourself coming with such force that your body rises off the table.

Then it's over. Ingrid is stroking your thighs gently and your body floats back. She places a cool sheet over you and tucks it in all around your body, from shoulders to toes, and you feel deliciously enveloped.

Before drifting off to sleep you look up. Ingrid smiles and asks in broken English, "Gut massage, no?" You smile back and say weakly, "Gut massage, yah!"

5

Covered by a Sheet

YOU COULD SEE nothing at all. It was totally dark. Not even the tiniest glimmer of light was able to get through the windows they had sealed so tightly. The darkness of the night outside was noontime sun compared to this black room.

You couldn't remember why it had seemed so important to be part of this group with their secret rites and peculiar behavior. You knew vaguely that it involved some sex things, and you were a bit afraid. But you had agreed. You had to break out of your shell. You were so inhibited sexually that it made you uncomfortable even to play with yourself! You were always afraid someone was watching—a thought that both turned you on and scared you.

When Marsha had asked you to come and meet some of her friends, your stomach knotted with anxiety. You hesitated only for an instant though and said yes before she could ask twice. Your curiosity was driving you beyond your neurotic inhibitions.

You had been blindfolded and carried, by how many people you didn't know, and placed on a bed. You had been stripped first and so as you lay there, you could feel the coolness of the sheet beneath you. Your blindfold had been removed, but the darkness was its replacement. Now you felt something lovely. A satin sheet was put over you. It had holes at your nipples and genitals. The rest of you was completely covered.

Click! A small light was turned on. Now you could see that the sheet was black, and this was a spotlight shining only on your pubic area. The heat of the bulb warmed you.

Suddenly a quiet but firm male voice said: "I'm going to fuck you, but I can't see your face and can't see who you are. You don't know who I am either. I'm just going to fuck you and fuck you until you moan and come."

As he spoke he climbed on top of you, and you felt the hardness of his penis at the entrance of your vagina. Although you had no preparation, and were not even lubricated you didn't dare object to his entry into your body.

He kept talking as he moved inside you with forceful thrusts.

"I don't give a damn who you are. You're just a cunt. A cunt for me to fuck."

It was so strange, but this total removal from any pretense of tenderness was getting you very turned on. You lay beneath the black sheet and received him. There was no embarrassment either. You didn't wonder about being watched, even though you knew the room was probably filled with people, all staring at the hole in the sheet which revealed your most private area. The blackness of that sheet was your protector—your safety. And it freed you.

You started to moan softly as he kept up his rhythm. Always fucking and always talking impersonally.

"That cunt will always be available to me, and I'll fuck it whenever I want."

Your body responded with unbridled lust. He seemed to grow harder as your excitement increased and as he pumped away you heard another voice—at first not even recognizing it as your own. Your breathing was noisy and you were saying, "Yes! Yes! More! Fuck me harder! Yes! Yes!" And then you were screaming, "Oh God yes, yes, faster, **FASTER!**" and suddenly you came. God, did you come! It never stopped. Only then did he pause for a moment, and you heard a loud sigh as he poured his hot seed into your clutching vagina.

And then the spotlight was turned off, and you felt yourself drift off to sleep, happy you had joined the club.

6

Neighbors

HAVING ONLY RECENTLY moved into the neighborhood, you don't know many people yet. But you're very eager to meet and make new friends. Your husband, David, has urged you to invite your downstairs neighbors up for a drink, and he wants you to be as nice as possible to them. You've promised to try to overcome your painful shyness and come out of your shell.

Supper is finished and Stan and Merle will be arriving any minute now. Just as you're looking over the living room one last time to make sure everything is in place, the doorbell rings. As you go to answer it, David puts some soft music on the stereo.

As your guests enter and admire your home, you can't help but notice how good looking they both are. Stan is about two inches taller than David, and even though he's wearing a long sleeved sports shirt, you can see how muscular his arms are.

Oh goodness, you're doing it again. Every time you meet a new man, you appraise him physically. You suppose it's because you really don't think David is all that handsome—even though you love him very much. But tonight you see that you're not the only one who's doing the looking. David has been openly staring at Merle's very large breasts which are barely contained under the skintight sweater she's wearing.

"How about a drink?" David suggests, and everyone agrees.

While he goes to get some ice, you can't help getting the feeling that these new friends are different from anyone else you've met so far. Each time you steal a glance at Stan, you're surprised to find that he's looking you over as well. You're flattered because although you're pretty, Merle is quite a knockout, and you wouldn't expect her husband to desire any other girl.

Soon you've settled into the comfortable living room. One round of drinks follows another until you're all beginning to loosen up. It's then that Merle suggests a game.

"Why don't we play strip poker?" she giggles.

You all laugh but she persists.

"Oh, *please* let's play."

You're a bit taken aback when David says, "Sure, why not?"

He gives you a meaningful look, since he knows this is something you would not want to do. But you've promised to try . . . And if he's willing to go along—well, so are you.

"Okay," you find yourself saying. And then you really can't back out—even if you wanted to.

David finds a deck of cards, and you arrange yourselves on the floor. The first hand is dealt and before long everyone has taken off a few bits of clothing. Shoes are discarded first, then belts. The men take off their shirts next and the girls their slacks. You are upset to realize how much the game is turning you on, and when you see Stan losing the next hand, you feel your breath catch, you're *that* eager to see what he looks like underneath his pants. He takes them off and his legs equal his arms in form. They are muscular but not overly so. He's really a fantastic-looking man. Merle giggles at Stan sitting there in his jockey shorts.

Soon you're all down to bras and panties and jockey shorts, and the next one to lose a hand will have to do quite a bit of revealing. It's David, and suddenly he's completely naked. You quickly look over to Merle who is not a bit shy about inspecting his crotch. She shows her approval by smiling broadly. (You silently wonder to yourself how this all got started!)

Stan loses a hand then and has to remove his shorts. You're disappointed at the size of his penis which seems so small. You had imagined him to be huge. You blush, embarrassed by your thoughts and you want to run out of the room. As if he senses this, David takes your hand and gives you a pleading look, and without speaking a word, you know he wants you to go on.

Merle loses next, and she takes particular relish in removing her bra. God! Her breasts almost jump out as she unhooks the back of her bra and they just stand there large and beautiful. Their only flaw is a round scar an inch above the nipple of the right breast which makes you think of a cigarette burn.

You're awfully envious, but you feel a strange desire to let everyone see how lovely your own breasts are—even though they are much smaller than Merle's. And so, when your turn comes, you slowly remove your bra to reveal your own firm breasts.

All at once, Stan puts his hand on Merle's breasts. You're unable to move and neither can David.

"Aren't they beautiful?" Stan asks.

"Well, yes, they certainly are," you both mutter, fascinated.

"How would you like to feel them?" he asks David, who gives you a quick look but then doesn't even reply. His hand shoots out and lightly touches her breasts.

"You can do better than that," Stan says.

David follows his lead. Soon he's nibbling away at her luscious chest, making her squirm with delight. But you don't have much time to watch for Stan is beside you and he's playing with your breasts. He seems to love them and he is touching and pulling your nipples, which take very little time to respond. You lose whatever reluctance you might have had and just lie on the floor enjoying it. You look out of the corner of your eye and see David moving his hands all over Merle's body. Instead of being jealous, you find yourself excited at the sight and you're urging Stan to do the same. Before long, Stan is all over your body with his hands, his tongue, his penis.

He's above you and now his penis has grown enormously.

Its flaccid size was deceptive. Erect it's almost the same six inches as David's. You are so wet, he slips in without a problem. Stan moves slowly at first, until you adjust to his rhythm. Then you find yourself pulling him closer to you and whispering for him to move faster.

David is doing the same to Merle, who's enjoying it as much as you. You feel an uncontrollable urge to share your delight with her, too, and you lean over and kiss her on the mouth. She returns your kiss and the two of you continue kissing while you're being made love to by your husbands. You reach out and touch her breasts and she reciprocates. Soon the four of you are wrapped up in each other's pleasure. The men stop for a moment to sit back and watch you.

Your fondling of one another has obviously excited the men. David now turns you around and begins to screw you doggy fashion. Merle massages your clitoris, just as if drawn to it by a magnet. Stan is in front of you with his penis staring you in the face. He pushes it into your mouth and begins to move it in and out just as he had done to your vagina. David is staring, and his excitement grows and grows until he's pounding away at you like a jackhammer. You know he's about to come; he can't contain himself. He squirts his hot liquid into you. It seems like quarts. You can't remember him ever coming this much. He sinks to the floor, out of the action but watching the rest of you.

Stan keeps his penis in your mouth and now has your head in his hands so that even if you want to move away, you can't. His eyes are closed while he endlessly pounds himself into you. Then he too comes. His semen pours into your mouth until you can't swallow any more. When the last milky drop has spurted into you, he lies down too.

Merle silently moves over to you, pushing you down onto your back and moves her head to your dripping bush. The cum from David is still in you, but she doesn't flinch. She goes at it as if it were a butterscotch sundae. She licks around your vagina and clitoris and sucks away at you, lapping up every drop of cum. All the time she's playing with her own clitoris, getting herself as excited as you are. You reach down and guide your friend's head so that her tongue will flick over those spots which give you the most pleasure.

Soon you feel your body tense and you want to put off coming as long as you can, but you know you can't hold back any longer. Merle is right with you, bringing herself to the same level with her hand. You feel yourself losing control. You are aware of every part of your body—all your muscles working towards this climax. You hold her head to you until she flicks your clitoris one last time, and you gasp as an orgasm like none you've ever had rushes over you. Yours has set hers off and she sighs with pleasure. Your body shakes and goes into spasms, and she keeps licking at you until you feel the relaxation coming on like a diver drifting to the surface of the water after the thrill of a perfect dive.

The four of you exchange looks before sinking into the arms of your mates. You're happy about the new friends you've made.

7

At the Office

YOU'VE HAD THIS job for several months. You're an efficient secretary who enjoys her work, although sometimes you wished the men in the office wouldn't ogle your voluptuous figure so openly.

You've even caught your boss, Mr. Marshall admiring you. You ignored it, but secretly you think he's cute.

One day, while you're sitting at your computer, Mr. Marshall walks over to your desk. He says he's come to look for something he left in your bottom drawer the night before.

"Don't bother to move," he says as you start to get up. "Keep on working, I'll manage."

So you go back to your typing. He bends down and riffles some papers in the drawer. All of a sudden, you feel his hand on your ankle. Was it an accident? It doesn't move — it stays there, as if waiting for some kind of response. After an uncomfortably long pause, you feel his hand creep up your leg and then stop again. You decide you like it. Your silence is his signal to go further. You're totally composed. No passerby would have guessed it wasn't business as usual.

Before very long his hand is between your legs playing against your panties, over the lips of your cunt. You don't skip a letter typing in a determined effort not to attract attention in the office. But your eyes are closing and your breathing starts to quicken.

Now he's managed to reach your wet cunt and has begun inserting his fingers in and out, very slowly. You try not to give a clue to the below-desk activity, but it's getting more difficult. He increases the tempo now, moving his fingers quicker and quicker. You reach in back of you, searching for his penis. He helps you by unzipping his fly. Your fingers wrap around his shaft, and you start playing with him. You're still facing the opposite direction, typing with one hand. You jerk him rapidly, and inside your cunt, his hand keeps time with yours. Your clit is as hard as his penis.

It only takes a little more of his rubbing before you have a very enjoyable orgasm. In a moment he zips up his pants, stand up, and walks back into his office. You smooth down your skirt and return your full attention to the letter you're working on. No one in the office is the wiser.

Brother and Sister

FOR MANY YEARS you and your brother have had separate bedrooms, but tonight there are weekend guests and you have to share his room. You both get undressed quietly, hidden from each other, and crawl under your respective sheets. The room is dark, but you know from his breathing that your brother is very much awake.

"Warren," you call.

"Yes," he whispers.

"Are you asleep?"

"No," he says. "Are you?"

You giggle a little bit at this stupid conversation and you feel a certain warmth running up and down you as the image of your brother's firm body begins to give you all sorts of naughty, but sexy, ideas.

"I'm cold," you say. "Is it always so cold in here?"

"Sometimes," he answers.

"Warren, why don't you come here and warm me up?" you suggest coyly.

"How do you mean?"

"Well, if you just get in with me under the covers, our bodies will warm each other up.

"Okay," he says.

Warren climbs to the bunk below him where you are. The two of you lie still as minutes tick by. You keep your bodies from touching, scarcely daring to breathe. Then, pretending you're asleep, you turn and let your hand fall on the top of his pajama pants. Your finger is on the string. Slowly you move onto his fly and down. There's movement and you know that he's responding. In a very, very slow way, your hand reaches further down and the back of your fingers rest against his stiff penis. You wrap your fingers around it. It's long and thin and hard.

His only response is a muffled sigh.

Not taking your hands off his penis, you roll around and kiss him. You kiss him again and he wraps his arms around you. You are both panting now.

With your other hand, you pull the string and start to take his pants slowly off. When you find your face at his cock, you stick out your tongue and lick the very tip. Almost instantly, white semen shoots out.

When there's no more, you take a tissue from the night table and dry him off. His penis has shrunk to about an inch and a half, so you lean down to lick his balls. He lays there as if nailed to the bed, not moving, but again he hardens.

"Hey, baby brother," you tease, "you hungry? Would you like something good to eat?"

You guide his head to your pussy. He buries himself in it and you thrust your head to his cock. You are eating with the eagerness of kittens lapping up bowls of milk. When it's too much to stand, you push yourself around and sit up on his cock. It fits so neatly into you. As your bodies blend, he comes, groaning. You reach forward cupping his face with your hands and kiss him passionately. You know now you have a new lover, and it's all in the family.

9

Domination

IT HAS BEEN several weeks since you've last seen Steve. You'd been arguing with him. He insisted that he have absolute control over you, and you refused to accept such chauvinistic crap. But now as he starts to undress you, you only look forward to enjoying yourself in bed — it's been so long since the last time.

He unhooks your dress, pulls it down over your hips, and lets it drop to the floor. You step out of it. He pulls down your panties and you stand in front of him, completely nude. The large nipples on your soft breasts are already erect in anticipation of the delicious love-making you know will follow.

He leads you to the bed, and you lie down on your back, your body tingling with excitement. He stands above you, next to the bed, and runs his fingers slowly down your body. Soft music plays in the background. He begins to suck on your nipples, and you get very hot. He runs his fingers between your legs, and you feel your cunt begin to lubricate. One finger brushes against your labia, and your legs open wider. He slips his finger inside the yielding wetness. You're ready for him.

You reach up and feel the weight of his balls in your hand. He's already erect. You begin to play with his penis slowly. Then you crane your head and start to suck on him. He lies down next to you, and you can hardly wait for him to come into you.

"Wait a minute," he says suddenly. "I'll be right back." He walks into the next room while you're left squirming on the bed. To say the least, you're surprised when he returns with a girl and a guy—people you've never seen before. You pull the blanket around yourself, puzzled and confused.

Steve yanks away the cover. "Don't touch it," he commands. "Just lie there the way you are." You ask what this is all about, and he says, "I told you—you're mine and I can do anything I like with you."

Then he orders you to play with his penis. His tone is frightening, so you obey. You barely touch him, and he is hard again. He sticks it into your mouth, and you suck it. You're quite aware of the two people standing there, watching, while you suck off Steve. You want to pull away, but he has your head locked to his body. He's moving in and out of your mouth. Then he withdraws and tells the man to take off his clothes. The woman undresses, too, and each of them stands next to the bed, neither having said a word. Steve asks the man if he'd like to fuck you, and you recoil in horror.

"Steve, you can't do this to me."

"Watch, and you'll see how I can do it to you," he replies coolly.

Steve holds your arms and the woman holds your legs while the stranger mounts you. His penis is still flaccid. Steve tells him to move up to your face so you can suck him into erection. He straddles you. You can't escape, so you start sucking. It quickly hardens and then he moves down again, forcing himself into your vagina so roughly that it hurts.

At first you squirm, trying to expel this unwanted object. But as his thrusts continue, you respond to this stranger. You soon are eagerly meeting his strokes. You never thought you could respond like this to anyone but your lover, but here you are, your body working faster and faster to keep up with the stranger's passion. When the girl releases your legs, you don't even try to escape.

She comes alongside you and begins sucking on your

nipples. This gets you even more excited. While she sucks on one breast, Steve is working on the other. You're vaguely aware of you inability to discern which mouth is male and which female. All the while, the stranger is screwing you, and you are matching his pace.

The girl climbs up and places her hairy bush right at your mouth. You want to turn away but Steve commands you to eat her. He grabs your head and slaps you roughly in the face. Once again you are afraid of him and so you begin to lick her. You start slowly and delicately, not knowing what to do at first. You decide to pretend you're actually doing this to yourself. You stroke her clitoris and it tenses. You probe her vagina, first moving slowly, but as you hear her passionate mewing sounds, you go faster and stronger. You're surprised at how well you seem to be pleasuring her. All the time the stranger is fucking you.

Suddenly she gasps and you realize that she's at an orgasm. It's such a weird feeling to know that you could make another woman climax just as Steve has made you come so many times. In a few moments it's over and she rolls off you to the side, lying there contented.

At this point the man takes his penis out, and Steve turns you around to fuck you doggy fashion. The stranger moves up to your face and shoves his stubby cock in your mouth.

You're totally caught up in the excitement and respond without thinking at all. You become aware of the girl's fingers on your clitoris, playing with you, trying to make you come. As her hand rubs in a circular pattern the feelings begin. She then rubs each side of the shaft, pulling the skin around the clit taut. She alternates these motions for a while as it rises higher and higher. You have no control at all. As you come, gasping and squealing, Steve fucks you faster and faster, making you feel as if your orgasm could last forever.

Finally Steve shoots his hot cum into you. You want to

stop everything now, your body aches with exhaustion, but the stranger holds your mouth around his cock. He keeps pumping into your mouth until, with one last thrust, he spills himself into you as you try to swallow it as fast as it pours out.

After this you won't question Steve's power over you.

10

A Dog Day

WHEN YOU PEEKED out the open porch door that hot summer night, you thought you saw your cousin Joey off to one corner of the front yard. You were about to shout hello when his activity suddenly came into focus. He was bent down on one knee, petting your dog, King. But it was more than casual attention he was paying to King. He had one hand underneath the dog, who was standing absolutely still. You couldn't see all of it right away, but then you did. He was playing with King, pulling at the dog's penis, and even muttering "Good dog, good dog."

Ugh! You wanted to yell at him to stop. At the same time, you were strangely fascinated. You couldn't take your eyes away. It didn't take very long. In a moment King's body lurched slightly, and you thought you saw something whitish shoot out in front of him. When it was over, you pulled yourself back to your senses and did call out.

"Joey, you should be ashamed of yourself," you reprimanded. "If you touch King again, I'm going to tell mama."

Joey was caught off guard but quickly regained his poise and took the offensive.

"Oh yeah?" he challenged. "Well I knew you were there watching. And if you say anything, I'll just say you put me up to it." You couldn't come back with an answer, and your hesitation encouraged Joey to jump ahead in a more confidential tone. "You want to try doing it? It's fun."

"I think it's disgusting," you answered and began to walk away.

"No, it's fascinating," he said, using your word as if he had read your mind earlier. "King has an enormous thing, and it's all red. I'll bet you never even took a good look at it."

When again you said nothing, he went on with his pitch, describing how he did it whenever he could. Sometimes King lay on his back, other times he'd sort of try to "mount" Joey's leg, and still other times he'd just stand there like he had that night.

You felt yourself growing flushed. Joey noticed that the talk was obviously turning you on.

"Come on," he said persuasively, "you don't have to do it, but why not watch?"

So you followed Joey—this time farther away from the house, where nobody could see you. It was late and everyone was probably asleep. You hadn't been able to fall asleep and that's why you had just grabbed your light cotton robe and put it on to go downstairs to get some cool air. Joey led you and King to a secluded corner of the yard, behind a tree.

"Here King," Joey beckoned in the same voice you'd heard earlier. As King came closer, he reached in front of the dog again and started pulling and massaging him. You couldn't see very well, so you bent lower. Joey continued for a few moments and then reached for your hand and put it on the emerging, glistening, red penis. You tried to pull away, but he held you firmly and moved your hand up and down as more and more of the dog's penis came out. You were surprised and revolted by its feel, but you couldn't take your hand away. As you moved it the dog responded with quick jerky motions. In a moment he shot again and some of the cum landed on your robe.

"Oh, that's horrible!" you cried. "Now what am I going to do? I'm covered with it!"

Joey suggested you take off your robe and let it dry off, but you explained that you had nothing on underneath.

"So what?" he said coyly. "We're cousins. . . .

You felt silly being there, and annoyed with yourself, but you took off your robe and lay it down. You didn't hear Joey come up behind you, but you did feel his hands on your breasts. He was kissing your neck and though you tried to break loose, he was much stronger than you. You threatened again to tell your mother, but he only laughed and said that it would be his word against yours. And besides, what were you doing there anyway? And what was that dog stuff doing on your robe?

You were angry and frustrated—and trapped by Joey. As he held you tightly, he played with you until you felt your body relax and respond. He moved his hands down now and touched between your legs. It was wet. You both knew that jerking off King had gotten you all worked up.

Joey was pressing against you, and you felt him bulging in his pants. He unzipped his fly, took out his cock, and started brushing your naked rear with it as he kissed your neck and fondled your breasts. Your body relaxed more and more. He pushed you down so you were on all fours and started whispering, "That's a good girl, that's good ..in the very tone he had used with King!

All of a sudden you felt the tip of his hot cock at your vagina. You were so wet, it slid in quickly. He groaned as if in agony and started pumping. You returned his thrusts and even increased their speed.

You felt King sniffing around you, but you were too involved to try to figure out what he was doing. Joey said something, ordering King away. The dog had been trying to mount him. King kept coming back though, apparently ready for more. There was no getting rid of him. Joey pulled out of you, and as you were about to stand, you felt his strong hand push you back into your position on all fours. Then you felt something furry at your back. You started to scream, "No, no. . . ," but Joey put one hand over your mouth. You tried to get away, but Joey was just too strong. You heard that soft voice again, "Nice King, that's a good boy . . .," and then he inserted the dog's penis into you! You screamed again in revulsion, but the sound was muffled by Joey's hand.

King was firmly implanted in you and his paws were up on your buttocks. He was moving furiously. You were disgusted. But that feeling gave way to surprise as you found yourself moving back and forth with the dog. Your body couldn't help it! The dog's penis was in you and it felt good. Joey watched in amazement, and when he released his grip, you didn't try to escape, you were too much into it.

Joey moved around to stand in front of you. He pushed his stiff cock into your mouth and you took it greedily. He worked your mouth as King worked you. Suddenly you felt King shooting and lurching into you. You were very excited now and you started to come. Then Joey too exploded, into your mouth. You swallowed as much as you could while the rest dribbled out.

Later, in bed, you pulled the covers tightly around you. As you fell into a deep sleep, you wondered whether all of those incredible things had really happened, or whether it had been a dream.

11

Threesome

WHEN JUNE CALLED and asked if she might drop by for a while that evening, you didn't want to say no, especially since it had been a while since you'd last seen her. But you didn't really want to say yes, either. Bob was on his way over and you'd looked forward to an evening alone with him. But you never could say no to a friend. Now she was on her way and you were brooding about it when Bob arrived.

You greeted him with a long passionate kiss, and his response made you even sorrier that June would be there soon. When you told him there'd be company that evening, his smile faded and he looked quite disappointed. But then an impish grin appeared on his face.

"Well, maybe we can talk her into a threesome," he said.

"I don't think I'd like that," you replied, hurt. "Besides, June doesn't do those numbers. She and Wally are faithful and all that. . . . "

"Oh yeah?" Bob smiled more broadly. "I'll bet I can change her mind."

All at once the evening's scenario had changed and you felt tense and uncomfortable. You were responding jealously, but you had only yourself to blame for screwing the evening up.

You were sipping a drink when the bell rang again. You went to greet June feeling very uneasy and not very happy.

"Hi," she said, "so we finally get together." And then her eyes went to Bob on the couch.

"Oh, I'm sorry—you didn't tell me Bob would be here. I shouldn't intrude. Perhaps we should make it another time?"

"Don't be silly," Bob said, jumping up and coming forward. "Have a drink." And he pushed a gin and tonic into her hand.

It must have been the liquor, because after another couple of drinks, your tension seemed to disappear and you forgot about wanting June to go away. You were loose and a little giggly—and determined not to show your jealousy over Bob's interest in your friend.

"I can't stay very long," June said.

"Wally is home baby-sitting. He just sort of gave me some 'time off.' "

Bob moved so that he was between you and June, and soon had his arms around you both. June was looking at him quizzically. Bob pulled you closer to him and kissed you very long and hard—but didn't release June. When you parted she was flushed, and there was an awkward silence He leaned over to kiss her, too, and she obliged him by turning her head so all he got was her cheek. Bob pretended to be drunker than he was and demanded a "real" kiss. June again said something about leaving, but stopped in midsentence. Bob had turned on his "hurt" look. She gave in and allowed him to kiss her, lightly at first, but as you watched, you could see a slight change. Her body relaxed a bit, and soon she really was returning his kiss.

"Yummee!" Bob exclaimed when it was over.

"I guess I'm getting drunker than I realize," she managed to say lamely before Bob pulled her to him and kissed her again, this time letting his hand drift down to her breast area. You were amazed she didn't stop him. You saw his hand pass lightly over both breasts again and again and it was obvious she was beyond resisting.

In your discomfort you went for another round of drinks. It was quiet for a while. Then Bob began saying how he would love to have June join you in bed. She looked flabbergasted but not appalled. He told her how much he liked kissing her and how he'd love to fondle her body. June seemed hypnotized by all this flattery and was unable to decide whether to run or to go on listening. Bob finally remembered you were there too, and he turned and pulled you to him. You were on his knee when he started his pitch again.

"I think the two of you have such beautiful bodies," Bob went on. "June, take a look at these breasts!" He quickly pulled up your blouse to reveal them. You always felt self-conscious and embarrassed because they were so large.

She couldn't take her eyes from them. "How beautiful they are!" she said in a husky whisper. You were startled to recognize a trace of envy in her voice.

Bob began to kiss and nibble at your nipples which, though small, were extremely sensitive. Your eyes closed as you felt yourself falling through the sky. June was mesmerized. Bob stopped long enough to pull her blouse off, and you and June were facing each other, nude from the waist up. Bob started taking turns fondling each of you and neither of you dared to move. You merely sat there, and you were sure June shared your surprise and excitement.

But guilt got the best of June and she started to rise. "I *really* should go . . .," she said weakly, but Bob pulled her down again and kissed her—this time using one hand to stroke her breasts while the other fondled you. You were fascinated, watching their lips meet. Their mouths barely touched and you could see Bob's tongue reach into June's eager mouth. Hers met his and went deep into his mouth, exploring avidly. Soon he turned to kiss you. He moved his hand down your body and traced an invisible circle about your navel. An electric shock seemed to jolt you. June watched as Bob opened your pants and removed them. He separated your legs and had you lie on the floor in front of the couch.

"Have you ever examined another girl's bush?"

June couldn't reply, she waited numbly for whatever would follow.

"Look how lovely it is," Bob went on, "how wet she is, and how it opens to my touch." As he spoke in a low, soothing tone, he started playing very lightly between your legs, and you were sticky and wet with excitement.

"Now you do it," he directed June. She hesitated. Bob took her hand and moved her fingers in imitation of his own. She was unable to move away, even after he took his own hand from on top of hers. Mmm . . . it felt lovely, you thought vaguely.

You felt yourself being drawn into another world, not caring who was playing with you. It felt good and that's all that mattered. You heard June breathing heavily over you, and you saw Bob get behind her and remove the rest of her clothing without her seeming to be aware of it. You reached out to return the good feelings to her, and she moved so that you could reach her more easily. Soon the two of you were in the "Sixty-nine" position, touching, exploring, and you wanted to know how she would taste.

You moved her legs so they were over you, just as you had done hundreds of times with Bob. After a brief pause June's body was against your face. She tasted .. . almost sweet. And the textures were smooth and slippery, but lovely. You moved your tongue the way Bob did to you, and June let out a sigh indicating she was thoroughly enjoying it. Her body met your tongue and she began to kiss you as well, duplicating your own gestures. God! It felt so good. Was it possible that she could be better than Bob?!

Bob watched for a while before undressing. He stood over the two of you. He played with himself and as you cracked your eyes, you saw his erection hovering above you. He leaned down and moved your bodies slightly pulling June off of you. He entered you in the mouth and started to move in and out very slowly.

He suddenly withdrew and went into June, who lay next to you. She gasped in her excitement. He moved around in her and then he began alternating, first plunging his penis in her vagina and then in your mouth—from one to the other. Her taste was on his penis and you found yourself hungrily licking him clean only to be waiting for the next time he left her body to enter your mouth.

Then Bob concentrated on fucking June and you became very excited watching them. You ached for release but they were too wrapped up in themselves to be aware.

You decided you had to do something to relieve all the tension which had been building up during this scene. You reached down between your legs shyly. You began to massage your clitoris and tried to focus only on the pleasurable feelings which started coursing through you. It was difficult. You felt awkward in front of them. You had never before masturbated in front of another person. The playing started to work and you lost your self-consciousness as the glow came on.

When you climaxed, it was abrupt and not as explosive as you had hoped it would be. But your body was fulfilled nevertheless.

As you started to sink into a cloud of relaxation, you felt fingers reach for your clit. It was Bob who had been watching you. He helped to extend your pleasure by playing with you and your body shuddered with delicious spasms.

When you had been sated, Bob moved and pushed his penis into your mouth and pumped furiously. In a moment he filled that orifice with hot semen. He turned then to June and began to lick at her noisily, and she too climaxed with a violent shiver.

Later, Bob and you drove June home. No one talked, instead choosing to relive the evening privately. You wondered hopefully if there would be a next meeting of the threesome.

12

The Widow Meets a New Friend

YOU HAD SAID no so many times that when Marion called and invited you to dinner to meet a "nice widower," you felt you couldn't beg off again. She meant well, even though you thought she was rushing you into meeting people before you were actually ready.

All your friends were after you. A year of mourning was enough, they said. How could you try to explain to them? You had been married for more than thirty years when Al died. You had known only one man for all those years. It was very difficult even to *think* about meeting anyone new.

But you decided to accept the invitation and although you dreaded it as the day approached, it was something you had to do.

There were eight people in all. Marion, her husband, her sister-in-law and her husband, a neighbor and her boyfriend, and you. And, of course, the man they'd invited for you to meet, Phil.

When you glanced at him, he seemed to be almost as uncomfortable as you. That put you more at ease — at least he wasn't some sort of ogre. You guessed him to be a few years older and just a bit taller than you. You were happy to see he hadn't gone bald, and though he had a slight paunch, he seemed in good shape.

As time passed you relaxed even more. It wasn't until you had been at Marion's for nearly an hour, that Phil actually came over to talk to you.

"Hi," he said, shyly. "Marion always tries to throw people together. I guess she gave you the same routine she gave me."

"Well. . ." you started to reply.

"Oh, I don't mean she forced me to come," he added quickly. "As a matter of fact, now that I'm here, I'm glad I accepted."

You felt flattered and smiled. "I'm glad I came, too."

The evening passed quickly from that point on. Although Phil was technically "with" you, he didn't hang on or cling to you. You liked that. Dinner was delicious—Marion always loved to fuss and show off her culinary skills—and after coffee and dessert, everyone started leaving. Phil came near and suggested that he take you home. As you left together, Marion gave you a contented smile. Frankly, you were glad you had let Marion twist your arm.

Once you were in Phil's car, though, the awkwardness returned. You were filled with feelings of guilt as if you were being unfaithful, somehow, to your late husband. Even though you knew that was ridiculous, you couldn't push those feelings aside. Phil seemed to sense this and he tried to put you at ease.

"I know just how you're feeling. Is this the first time you've been with someone since your husband died?"

You looked at him, amazed that he was reading your mind.

He went on, "I felt the same way after my wife passed away. 'How could I do this to her?' But you know, corny as it sounds, life *does* go on, and you must go on, too."

He reached over and took your hand and gave it a squeeze, in a show of friendship. You let it rest in his while he drove. You felt at ease then and the conversation was more relaxed.

"Why don't you sit closer?" he suggested.

When you hesitated, he acted a bit hurt. Still he held onto your hand. He continued talking, but you silently hoped the ride would end soon. You were weary from the amount of energy this evening had taken. Even though Phil was nice, you yearned for the security of your own home.

When he pulled over to the curb in the middle of the next street, you were puzzled. "Look," he said, "I'd like to talk to you." You didn't know how to reply, so you just listened.

"You're a very nice woman, and I find you very attractive."

As he spoke you felt him pulling you towards him.

"Please don't," you started to say, but Phil went on.

"Aren't you lonely sometimes? I am. Why don't you just relax?"

Now you found yourself actively resisting, trying to push him away, but he was much stronger than you. He had you pressed against his chest in a moment.

When he reached abruptly for your breast, you were shocked.

"Don't do that!" you shouted. "I'm not ready for that."

"What the hell do you think I am," he asked, "some kid? I didn't want to take you home just to talk. . . ."

All attempts at conversation stopped.

Phil gruffly planted a kiss on your mouth, hurting you as he ground his lips against yours and forced his tongue into your mouth. You twisted your face away, but he quickly brought it back so that he could kiss you again. You wanted desperately to get out of the car . . . .

He reached again for your breast and pulled it roughly. With an effort he pushed you down so that you were lying with your head against the car door. He lifted himself quickly and lay on top of you.

With his body pressed against yours, you felt the hardness of his erection poking against you through the light material of your dress. With one hand he drew up your skirt and pulled your panties apart enough to let him insert his finger between your legs. You were astonished to discover how wet you were! All that talk and just meeting him had stimulated you without you realizing it. When he touched you, you started to tremble.

"Please don't," you whispered. When he continued, not

heeding you at all, you changed your request. "Please . . . be, be, more gentle. . .."

For a moment he stopped altogether and lifted his head so that you looked deeply into his eyes. He was able to see the sincerity of your plea. He realized that you were no longer asking him to stop—but just to be kind to you.

Immediately, he changed. He was no longer the gruff, hateful person he had become. He kissed you, again, but this time his lips barely touched yours. He kissed you over and over and you soon relaxed and began to enjoy it. Your lips parted to allow his tongue to enter. As it did, you used your own in response. Now his hands traveled down your body, exploring—not grabbing as before, but probing, discovering.

He brushed your nipples lightly and reached through the opening of your dress to touch your flesh. You reacted with soft murmurs of delight. When he reached between your legs this time, they opened without a struggle. He pulled off your panties.

He barely touched you with his fingertips and within moments you felt an orgasm rush over you. It was there and gone, leaving you limp. Phil opened his pants revealing a very hard penis. He entered you. It brought you to life again and as he pushed, you met each of his tender thrusts. He put his hands around your buttocks to hold you as close as possible. You clung to him as he moved in you.

Almost at once you felt another climax upon you. This one came from somewhere deep within you. As he continued moving, you felt it growing. From a tiny persistent glow, it became a flame, engulfing Phil as well as you. He sighed loudly—his body shuddered—and he relaxed on top of you.

After rearranging your clothing and gaining some composure, you rode the rest of the way to your home in silence. You left the car without inviting him inside. But you exchanged warm smiles. You knew you'd be seeing more of Phil.

13

Playtime in the Pool

ALL WEEK LONG you thought about Saturday night. You could hardly keep your mind on anything else. Finally Friday and five P.M. arrived. You put your paycheck in your purse, shut down your computer, and left work behind until Monday morning. Ahead was the weekend and the exciting, though somewhat scary, anticipation of Saturday night.

When Peter called to invite you, he was very specific. This was a swim party—but a special kind. A nude swim party.

You had heard rumors around town that Sharon held wild parties at her parents' house when they were away, but you never had known whether they were true. Well, now you did.

Peter's invitation threw you. You liked him so much, even though you had only dated a few times. And you hoped the feeling was mutual. But you couldn't believe he would ask you—a "nice" girl—to a party where everybody was going to take off their clothes. And your hesitation must have indicated these feelings.

"Oh, don't be silly," he kidded. "I'll keep an eye on you. Do you think I'd let anything bad happen to you?"

Oh, you *knew* he liked you. And now he was even telling you how much he wanted to protect you.

"But does anything else go on there?" you asked shyly.

"Aw, come on now . . ."

So all week you had butterflies in your stomach. You thought about the few dates with Peter. Although you had done some petting, you hadn't even undressed for him. This would be the first time he'd see you nude. (You hoped he wouldn't notice your heavy thighs.)

It actually excited you a little just thinking of it, but then you felt the color rush to your face in embarrassment and you tried to push the thought of you and Peter without clothes out of your mind.

Saturday. The hours seemed to be 120 minutes each, but at last the doorbell rang. You ran down the stairs past your mother, saying, "I'll get it Mom. It must be Peter."

When you opened the door, Peter had only a moment to wave hello — and goodbye — to your mother before you whisked him out.

You didn't talk in the car until you were almost halfway to Sharon's. Then you blurted out, "I don't know if I can go through with this, Peter."

"Look," he said, "I told you I'd take care of you, didn't I?" He sounded just a tiny bit annoyed.

He didn't say anything else after that, and you began to feel guilty. After all, if you didn't want to go, you could have broken the date earlier in the week. But the truth was you didn't want to take the chance that Peter would ask another girl.

"I'm sorry. I didn't mean anything. I know you'll be with me. I'll go along with it." And you watched him smile as he took your hand and drew you closer to him.

When you arrived at the party, you saw lots of familiar cars parked in front. Boy, you thought, if any of their parents knew. . . .

Then Peter led you behind the house to the pool where there were about a dozen people, all nude, of course. You knew practically everyone. You wanted to shut your eyes and stare all at the same time. You had never seen so many people without clothes on before. You stopped worrying about your figure when you noticed that most of these bodies were ordinary looking.

"Well, look who's here," you heard a familiar voice call. "Get out of those clothes, baby. I've been dying to see you."

You felt frightened suddenly and wanted to run, but then Peter's arm was on yours.

"Come on," he said in a low voice, "let's get something to drink first."

He handed you a glass. You started to sip, but decided to chug it down. You needed all the courage you could muster. It didn't take long to feel the relaxation alcohol offers.

"C'mon now," Peter said. "I'll help you." He pulled off your slacks and sweater. You felt everyone staring at you, so, before you could chicken out, you stepped out of your panties and unhooked your bra.

Then you quickly dove into the pool, trying to hide yourself beneath the water. Peter jumped in after you and drew you very close to him. You could feel the entire length of his body pressed against you. You hid your face in his shoulder, but he gently tilted it to his lips. He grew hard as he kissed you . . . and then there was giggling. You opened your eyes to find the entire party circling you, staring and laughing.

Someone said, "Okay, now for the initiation."

You looked frantically at Peter. He merely smiled and continued to hold you firmly in his arms.

"Take her up on the diving board, Peter."

"Yeah, we all want to see this."

You started to protest but the eager, mocking faces silenced you. You clung to Peter's hand as he took you to the board and ordered you to kneel at his feet.

"Please, don't do this to me," you begged, almost in a whisper.

"There's no way out," he said. "You'd better do what I say, or they'll only pick someone else to take my place."

Your eyes darted around once more, searching for an ally. There was none. All the warm feelings you had for Peter disappeared at that moment and were replaced by fury for him having brought you to this. You resigned yourself to whatever would follow.

Down you went to your knees and Peter came closer to you until his penis was in front of your mouth. He held you by your hair as he stuffed it in you. He began to move as his organ grew. It got harder and harder and you could hardly hold it all without gagging. Minutes passed. There was no noise now except the creaking of the board and sound of his penis thrusting in and out of your mouth. He stopped. Someone put a towel on the board and then Peter forced you to lie on it, just a few feet above the water, with all eyes on you.

He knelt between your legs, forcing them open. You had to hold onto him to keep from tumbling into the pool. Suddenly he penetrated you. It felt so hard and unexpected that you gasped. As he began a steady rhythm, you tried to lie there rigidly — not responding — to show him with your body how you hated him. But feeling his hardness inside you and his smooth body pressed against yours melted your resolve. Soon you were trying to take even more of him in you.

"That's it," he whispered. "Wrap your legs around me, honey." You did and now your bodies were like a unit, pumping and pumping. You didn't care that there were a dozen people cheering you on. The entire world consisted of Peter and you.

Now he quickened his stroke — almost uncontrollably. "I'm going to come," he shouted, and as he did, you felt his stickiness spewing into you. You felt lovingly toward him as you waited for him to rise.

You were about to get up, too, when you heard Peter — the Peter who had just made love to you — say, "Okay, who wants the honor of licking this out of her?"

Immediately another guy lifted himself from the pool and rushed to take up the offer. "No," you begged. "Please don't."

You tried to get up and run, but strong hands gripped you from under the board and held your hands and feet firmly.

Just before you closed your eyes, you saw Bill, a former classmate, put his head between your legs and with his fingers spread you apart. Oh! You would die if you could. But then all you felt was his tongue. It licked and lapped hungrily and thirstily drank Peter's juices. His tongue started to explore more persistently, playing with the insides of your vagina and teasing your clitoris. You kept your eyes shut tightly, hoping it would soon be over. But again your body betrayed you. You heard a low moan—it was you! Bill kept licking and teasing and licking some more as you felt your control leaving.

When he withdrew his tongue, your body pressed against his mouth for more. You heard him chuckle, "You like it, don't you?" Your only response was to force your vagina against his eager mouth.

They were still holding your arms and legs but you heard voices, "She's gonna come soon."

"Boy, does she get into it."

All at once it rushed over your body. You wanted only to lie there—to be left alone.

But it was not over yet. Bill pulled you up as you heard muttering. "Now the water jet."

"Yeah, now the jet." And you were back in the pool. You were so overcome by the events of the evening you could barely make out the faces all coming toward you. A dozen people were lifting you until your body was out of the water. They brought you to the shallow end where the newly filtered water was jetting out in a strong stream. They lowered you until only your head was above the surface. Your legs were positioned and pulled wide apart.

You felt a strong jet of water shoot into you. It was so strong, it was painful. You pleaded for them to let you go. Your pleas were ignored. Just when you thought you couldn't take any more, the pain dissolved into an urgent kind of pleasure. You felt the water rushing at you, inside you and all over your vagina, and you had absolutely no control. The water came with such force that you climaxed in seconds. And as it grabbed you, you felt your body rise out of the water totally overwhelmed, and you heard yourself scream in ecstasy.

The next thing you were aware of was lying at the side of the pool with a pair of arms around you. They were Peter's. He looked at you. "Welcome to the fold," he said.

14

Tutor and Student

I**T WAS SO** difficult making a living and it seemed impossible to catch up with expenses, much less get ahead. You ran frantically about and still had to give piano lessons after your nine-to-five job in order to just keep going. You had gotten so tired of those bratty kids, none of whom were the slightest bit interested in playing piano. Their parents were the ones who believed in giving every child some introduction to the "arts."

The only child you didn't really mind teaching was Henry. He apparently enjoyed learning and looked forward to your visits. It lifted your spirits and today had been such a downer you even were a bit more eager than usual to give him a lesson.

Henry answered the door.

"Where's your mother?" you asked, since she usually let you in.

"Oh, she had to go shopping," he replied. "Is it okay? Will you still teach me today?"

"Oh, of course, Henry," you answered. He was bothered by the possibility that you might leave. You followed him into the sunny room where the piano stood. He was such a shy boy and always so quick to blush. Your heart went out to him. You kept encouraging him, trying to give him more self-confidence.

He sat down at the piano and began with the scale which always started the lesson. You walked up and down behind him, keeping time and commenting gently as he practiced. Every so often you would lean over his shoulder and point to the music sheet. The session went on and he did other pieces. Once, when you leaned over him, you thought you saw his face flush.

As he played, you watched him from a distance. He had grown up in the year and a half you'd been visiting the house. He probably was about thirteen now and had put on weight and height. A young man was emerging from the boy. There was even a slight fuzz on his upper lip, which made you smile, imagining ahead to the years not too far in the future when he'd be shaving.

You had never looked at him as you did that day, and his attractiveness surprised you. He wore a polo shirt which revealed his arms and the hint of muscles. You were fascinated and couldn't take your eyes from them as his fingers moved across the keyboard. He glanced at you, your eyes met, and then you both looked away. You didn't understand why, but you were both a bit embarrassed.

You moved closer again, commenting on the playing and pointing over his shoulder. You moved closer still and leaned against his back slightly, as if to feel his body. What on earth were you doing? You retreated and tried to regain your composure. Henry faltered a bit and asked if you'd explain something. Once again you came over, this time placing your hand on his shoulder as you bent over him to answer.

All of a sudden you were very conscious of the fact that the two of you were alone in the house. You tried to keep your mind on the lesson, but it kept wandering back to his arms, and the budding mustache. . . . You sat down next to him and were slightly taken aback when you turned to see his eyes almost at the level of your own. As you talked you found yourself resting against him. His face was bright red now.

"Henry, I know so little about you," you found yourself saying. "Do you have any girl friends?"

His answer was an almost inaudible no.

"I don't know why not," you continued, "you're so nice looking and bright."

He didn't reply, but you wanted to reassure him. "Don't worry, you'll soon have plenty of girls."

Silence. Then he blurted out, "I wish you were my girl friend!"

He quickly turned his back to you, mortified. You were flattered but disconcerted. Of course you'd heard of students getting crushes on teachers. This was so sweet.

You turned him back around. "Now Henry, don't be upset," you said. "I'm very flattered that you like me. I like you, too."

"You don't really like me," Henry said. "You just think I'm a little kid."

"Well, you are young, but I don't think of you as a little kid."

Your words didn't seem to be helping, which made you want to kiss him. You did just that, brushing your lips slightly against his. You were shocked to find it felt so nice. And now it was your turn to blush. You tried to explain that lots of boys got crushes on their teachers. His head went to your shoulder, and you started stroking his hair. You both were silent now, but you felt you had opened this up and were responsible to see that he wasn't hurt.

"When you are older," you went on, "you'll kiss your girl friends like this" and to demonstrate you took his face in your hands and kissed him again. His eyes were closed and you found yourself kissing him over and over until he relaxed. Now you gently put the tip of your tongue into his mouth. He tensed for a moment, and then opened to receive it. His tongue met yours, and soon you were exchanging long sweet kisses.

As your tongues gently played, you moved your hand down his shoulders lightly to feel his young muscular arms. The jolt to your nervous system made your movements involuntary and he followed your every action. You placed his hands against your breasts. It took a couple of seconds before he had the courage to explore. You opened your blouse to let him reach inside. You took one hand and led it to your nipple. His hands were so soft and tender. Using your own hand, you taught him what to do. Your lips never left his.

You moved down his young body and felt him bulging through his pants. You placed your hands tenderly against him. He started breathing loudly. "It's all right," you whispered. "Try to calm down a bit."

You opened his pants and released his penis. It was larger than you would have expected and was standing up quite hard. You stroked him gently and whispered more words to him so he wouldn't climax immediately. You leaned down and took him into your mouth, licking him lightly all over. You felt below for the young fuzzy balls and tried not to hurt him or have him lose control.

Then you stood up, raised your skirt, and pulled off your panties. You let him see your hairy bush. He was mesmerized. You led his hand to it and showed him how to move his fingers to make you feel good. You were breathing quickly now yourself and wanted to feel that young penis in you. You told him to stand behind you. You turned so that your bare buttocks were facing him and your skirt was drawn up around your waist. You parted your legs and told him to move close to you and to put his penis into you.

When he did, you felt yourself open up to him. He moved in and out automatically, as if living out a fantasy he'd had many times. You realized he would come very quickly and you wanted to finish with him. You reached down to massage your clitoris, while whispering loving words of encouragement to him.

He was moving very quickly now and you felt yourself about to come. "Let go!" you cried. "Don't hold back any more." At that he came hot into you. It was amazing how much he came and this heat was soon followed by your own as your body went into the spasms of an orgasm. Soon he was limp, back on the bench, leaning against you.

You told him how wonderful it had been for you and how sweet he was, and as you did, you rearranged his clothing and your own. In a few minutes you heard the door open, and Henry's mother stepped into the room. You assured her that the lesson had gone well, and that he was certainly quick to learn.

15

Free Afternoon

I**T WAS A** crazy idea. But after washing dishes and wiping runny noses all day, you decided to do it. You called Barbara and suggested the two of you get a baby-sitter and put all four kids together in her apartment. "Then come up here for a break. Maybe we'll even treat ourselves to martinis."

At first she thought you were kidding. After all, it was three in the afternoon, lots to be done, dinner to think about. . . . But you persisted and she soon was convinced. The martini did it. "I can use a rest," she admitted. "Send the kids down, and I'll call somebody and be up right away.

You felt an excitement you didn't quite understand, but it turned you on, so you stayed with it. When the kids left, you put a pitcher and two glasses in the freezer. Before long Barbara was knocking on the "Well, here I am," she said. "I feel silly, but it's a fun idea to get away from everything once in a while. Where's my drink?!" You poured one for each of you. Before long you were both feeling no pain and just generally feeling relaxed and happy.

"You know what?" you said and blushed a little.

"No, what?" Barbara asked. When she saw you hesitate, she insisted, "Come on . . . you can't start something without finishing."

"Well, I was about to say that I've always thought you had really beautiful breasts."

"They droop a bit now, but they really were something before the kids," she replied. Now it was her turn to blush. She surprised you by saying shyly, "I've always kind of thought you had a very nice figure." This sent the two of you into embarrassed giggles. With the drink giving you courage, you moved toward her and asked, "What would happen if I did this?" You kissed her, just barely brushing your lips against hers.

She pulled away, very startled. She stared at you for a long time, but you didn't look away. Then she leaned forward and returned the kiss. You both smiled. Neither of you had ever kissed another woman, except for quick pecks on the cheeks of various and sundry female relatives. You felt the tip of her tongue reach into your mouth and you met it with your own. A tiny shock passed between you. Then your mouths were hungry and your lips and tongues were eager.

You reached out to pull Barbara closer to you and she offered no resistance. She came to you as if in silent agreement to follow your lead.

You helped her to the floor where you now lay beside one another on the soft shag rug. You kept kissing and holding each other and soon you were reaching out and touching her breasts. Wanting to feel them bare, you pulled off her sweater. Neither of you wore bras, so Barbara's large breasts were temptingly naked in front of you. You leaned down and licked one nipple. She sighed with pleasure. You followed no preconceived plan. You were totally into finding out all about her body.

You began sucking her nipples and pulling at them with your teeth. How lovely it felt to you, and Barbara obviously was enjoying it, too. She pulled your blouse up, separating the two of you for a moment.

You looked at each other after taking off the rest of your clothing. It was the first time you'd actually seen each other totally undressed, even though you had gone shopping together many times and shared dressing rooms. Now, neither of you could take your eyes off the other's nude body.

Barbara's fingers began exploring, tracing each of your

curves. She moved her smooth hands across your shoulders and to your breasts, leaning forward to kiss each one before moving down, along the contour of your hips. You had kept your body in good condition and felt proud as Barbara admired it. There was no jealousy in her eyes—just love and tenderness. She reached your hairy triangle and you couldn't help but notice that hers was much fuller than yours. It got you excited to see that luxuriant growth although except for the huge bush, she had very little body hair. She was the leader now and each of you were massaging the other's pubic area.

Soon you wanted to know more, so you slipped your finger inside her as she parted her legs to allow you entry. She was soaking wet and as her fingers entered your vagina, you realized you were, too.

She instinctively knew exactly how to probe and do your favorite things. She encircled your clitoris with two fingers, and every now and then inserted her middle finger deep into your vagina. Your hand imitated hers and you were soon moving frantically.

Next you positioned yourself so that your face was right at her bush and hers at yours. You wanted to taste her and put your tongue into her glistening cunt.

As you felt her tongue probing ever so gently, your only thought was how marvelous it felt. As she opened her legs wide to receive your mouth, you both seemed to be experiencing the identical pleasure. You licked up and down her crack and inserted your tongue as far as it would go. You moved to her clitoris and licked alongside it. Each time you moved your tongue away, she moved her body up to your face, telling you to do it again. You did. The delicious taste kept changing as she lubricated more.

You felt her mouth working on you and this took you up to an even higher plateau. She was sucking at your clit, pulling on it. It felt terrific. Every so often she would move her tongue back to flick past your ass. When she moved her tongue in and out of you, you felt your body responding to its tempo.

You were licking at her constantly now, and she was breathing in loud, fast pants. Her clit seemed to get even harder, and it all excited you so much that you felt yourself reaching your orgasm. She sensed this because as you came, she kept sucking and plunging her tongue inside you. This made you lick faster and harder at her and in a moment she joined you with her own orgasm. Her body kept trembling with each spasm and you worked your tongue until she gently pushed away your head.

As you rested beside each other you both agreed it had been a lovely way to spend the afternoon. . . .

16

Porno Movies

WHEN YOU ANSWERED the ad headed "Young Girls Wanted," you really hadn't been sure what it was for. "Impersonal Experiment" was all the paper had said.

Now you were in this rather antiseptic studio where there was nothing but glaring lights and whiteness. The total lack of shadow was disconcerting. You felt as if you had walked into an operating room. And the attitude of the man who met you at the door added to that feeling. Instructions were totally impersonal.

You were told you would be paid for one day's work. You were told where to disrobe. When you undressed and returned to the white room, you noticed several cameras. At first no one paid the slightest bit of attention to you, and since there was no place to sit or to lean, you found yourself standing, in the middle of all this activity, just waiting.

Soon a young, very handsome man came in, and he, too, was totally nude. He wouldn't look directly at you, but he seemed more at ease than you were, as if he'd been through this before. When the director came on the scene, things began to move more rapidly. A bed was brought in. Like everything else, it was stark. A white sheet covered it. Not a pillow or anything else broke up the bare effect.

"Now just lie down, you two," the director ordered.

Your partner followed instructions and you aped his actions.

"Start to play with her nipples," he said, and quite automatically, the fellow did. You just lay there and soon your nipples began to stand at attention.

"And you, pull at his penis," the director said to you.

At first you were a bit shy, but you had walked into this voluntarily, so you weren't going to back down now. You reached out and started stroking him. Before long, you were fondling and exciting each other, but neither of you looked directly at the other.

It was all so impersonal and strange, with the director calling his instructions, like a Fellini dream sequence.

"Move in camera Two a bit," you heard him say.

"Put your mouth over her left breast, please."

"Would you please insert your penis into the vagina now."

"A bit more quickly."

You were being fucked and yet it was as if you were sitting in a theater watching yourself on screen.

The weirdest thing was that in spite of all this detachment, you were getting aroused. You were breathing more audibly and you felt yourself lubricate. Through it all, the man on top of you, the man who was fucking you and playing with your breasts, never changed his blank expression.

It was like having a machine do it. You hated it and you hated him. You didn't know the first thing about him and yet you began to hate him. Hated him for not showing any emotion and for making you respond all the same. And yet, you had put yourself into this situation. . . .

You were panting now, but no one seemed to be aware of it. The director merely continued issuing his orders.

"Can we have that fellatio again, please?

How about trying to get into her ass?"

You were never consulted. You were being used as an instrument in some far-out orchestration. And still you felt your excitement grow. It reminded you of masturbating in front of a television set where the background sounds made no real difference to what was really going on.

As you got hotter and hotter, the director finally did notice and said, "It would seem she's about to come. We don't want to miss it, so please will you pull your cameras in tight."

His directions became more intricate and demanding.

"I want you to withdraw your penis, go down on her, and start lapping."

The stranger did this. You felt your clitoris responding with each lick of his well-practiced tongue.

"Slower, please" said the director. "This is quite good and we'd like to make it last as long as possible."

Your partner licked at your glistening hot vagina until you felt you would burst. Just as you were about to fly apart, he stopped, making your excitement subside. Your heart was pounding fast. You felt that you would pass out. Nothing could feel this intense for so long.

You found yourself literally gasping, so loud that the director responded, "I think we'd better let the poor girl get it off."

Your partner took his cue. He brought you slowly along and once again you felt yourself responding. You were moaning and almost begging. His tongue didn't stop this time. Your climax began to rise again. You knew that it wasn't going to be cut off again.

All the while the cameras pointed at you, your vagina, your face, the two of you. And all the time he lapped at your cunt.

With one last lick of his tongue it happened. Your whole body exploded. And then he began his licking again as your orgasm kept coming. Finally it stopped, and your body was at peace.

But before you had even a moment to rest, you heard the director's voice, "Well, we'll stop for a break now. After coffee bring in the next couple to join these two."

17

Bondage in a Gay Bar

YOU ARE BEING blackmailed. It's as simple as that. Four months ago when you had a brief affair with Tom, you never would have dreamed that now he would be threatening to tell your husband unless you went with him to some sort of erotic happening.

Your marriage was shaky enough without this. Sam and you had been on the verge of divorce many times but now things seemed to be working out. If he found out about the affair with Tom, the marriage would be over. You could only hate Tom for his betrayal of what you'd thought had been a lovely interlude in both your lives.

You met him at his apartment, having given Sam a story about visiting your friend Janet for the evening. Naturally you had to confide in her, even though sketchily, in case she needed to cover.

And so now you were on your way, and you didn't even know to where. You only knew you'd give anything to be home with Sam. You looked at Tom sitting behind the steering wheel and tried to figure out why you ever became involved with him. He wasn't handsome; actually his features were very rough, more like a guy who works outdoors than behind a desk. His build was okay but nothing special. You suppose you had been ripe for an affair, being so unhappy at home. And Tom had a certain magnetism—a persistence that few people, men or women, could resist.

He pulled the car to the curb. It was a rough neighborhood.

He led you silently to the bar with its garish neon sign flashing on and off. After sitting down at a table and ordering drinks, you looked and were startled to see there were mostly women dancing with women. Then you surveyed the room and saw that most of the tables were occupied by women. There were only a few men.

You had been brought up in a rather strict household and although you had heard about gay women, you had never seen one. Even if you had been more worldly, you would have never guessed, passing most of these girls on the street, that they were any less straight than you. Some were masculine looking, but it was more surprising to see the feminine types.

You asked Tom to take you home, but he only smiled and said, "Relax, honey, this party is just beginning."

You felt yourself turn cold and frightened.

As the evening went on, you drank and danced a bit. You couldn't see the point of Tom bringing you to this place. You kept looking at the women together and felt repelled by it all. You couldn't explain your reaction, but you just couldn't bear the thought of girls putting their arms around each other like men and women were supposed to.

After a while there were indications that the floor show was about to start. A woman dressed exactly like a man—suit, tie, short hair—came to the microphone and said, "Good evening ladies and gentlemen," and the audience giggled at the inside joke.

"Tonight we have a special event for the club. We have a debut."

Suddenly the spotlight swung around the room until it stopped at your table. You were totally confused. But then Tom was pulling you by the arm and leading you up to the stage. The women were applauding. The MC went on, "Our good friend Tom has brought a new young lady to be initiated into our way of entertainment."

You tried to ask Tom what was going on. "You just do what you're told," he interrupted, "and you won't get hurt. And your husband won't find out about this either." Just then some music began playing. You tried to look composed as you said, "I'd like to leave." The MC and Tom laughed.

Four girls came onto the stage. They were very tall and all naked. Their breasts were enormous, and they held what looked like shackles in their hands. Next a large table was brought out, and before you knew it, you were being held by the girls and your clothes were being taken off. You screamed and begged them to let you go. You began to cry, feeling completely lost and helpless. But nothing stopped them and no one paid any attention to you. The girls finished removing your clothing and carried you to the table. Now you knew what the shackles were for. Your hands and ankles were attached to the table so that you could not get away.

The music was louder now and one of the girls began to pull at your nipples. She pulled very hard, hurting you. Another one opened up your legs so that your vagina was completely visible to the audience, which had begun to cheer. They yelled out comments and directions to those on stage. The show was apparently underway.

The third girl went between your legs and opened them so wide you thought you'd be torn apart. You screamed again. This was something that you had never done, even with your husband, and here you were being violated by this woman. She went on as if deaf, paying no attention to your screams. She licked harder and harder, inserting her tongue into you like a penis, and darting it in and out. You shut your eyes tightly and lay there as the tears rolled down your face.

The last girl pushed away the one licking you. "That's no way to do it," she said. "I'm sure she'll like this better." She took over the position between your legs. She licked very gently, as though she truly didn't want to hurt you. You felt your body relax a bit. You thought that this one, at least, would not harm you. She kept lapping and exploring with her tongue, and you were shocked to feel your body getting aroused. Suddenly your vagina became very wet, and you could tell your clitoris was responding to the steady rhythm of her gentle tongue. All at once your body became rigid and you felt yourself come in a quick spasm. My God, how could this happen? You hated what was going on, and yet you'd had an orgasm. How ashamed you felt.

But before you could dwell on it, you saw a line of girls, all of them naked, getting ready to take their turns at you. One by one they licked at you. Some of them played with your nipples. It must have gone on for hours.

Finally, one girl, instead of going down on you as the others had, climbed up and straddled your face so that her vagina was right at your mouth. "Eat me!" she commanded. You turned your head, feeling only revulsion. "Eat me!" she repeated, this time slapping your face. You did.

At first you just touched your tongue to her very lightly, but she pulled your head hard against her. At the same time another girl was going down on you, and you felt your body coming round again. You began to lick the girl above you in imitation of the one at your vagina. You did everything you felt being done to you.

You were surprised that the taste, which you had feared, was not unpleasant. It was unusual, but after a moment it didn't turn you off so much. You began licking very quickly, and you felt her clitoris harden against your tongue just as yours had. A small thrill ran through you, totally confusing you. But you had turned on another person, and even if it was a woman—it excited you.

She loosened her hold on your face and very soon she moved her vagina against your tongue in such a way that you knew she must be about to come. You kept licking at the same pace, not daring to change it. Suddenly she had an orgasm and her body relaxed against you. As she got down from her perch, the girl tonguing you increased her tempo until you were again at the point of coming.

But she then stopped. You felt your body straining to meet her mouth, wanting her to continue. Then you felt something being inserted into you and realized that it was a dildo. It was very large and much harder than a penis. It completely filled you. She moved it in and out very roughly until you begged her to stop. She waited a moment, then continued the in-and-out movement. Her head was down again, licking your clitoris until you felt an orgasm rising out of your well.

Again she stopped. This time you felt something smaller being inserted into your anus. You did scream this time, the pain was so great. She used the two dildoes on your anus and your vagina until you thought you would pass out. And once again she put her head down to minister her lickings, but now she couldn't stop you. Your body went on and exploded with an overwhelming climax as the tip of her tongue barely touched you. You felt your vagina and anus contract around both dildoes as you went into spasm after spasm.

And finally it was over. You lay there as your clothing was put on. The music started again (when did it stop?) and Tom helped you to your feet. You could barely stand. He almost carried you to the car and drove you home in silence. As you entered your house, you saw Sam sitting in front of the television set.

"Have a good time, honey?" he asked.

"Not bad," you said, as you climbed the stairs to bed.

18

Nude on the Therapist's Knee

YOU WERE SO uptight these days that you always seemed on the verge of jumping out of your skin. You wanted to break out and free yourself emotionally, but you were having such a hard time. Lately, every therapy session was the same. You kept telling Doctor Simon that you wanted to "open up" and he kept urging you to.

"Just do it," he'd say.

"But what should I do?" you'd counter.

"Well, free yourself completely, be like a child."

Being like a child to you meant running naked in a forest.

"Well," he said, "for want of a forest we could turn the consulting room into a substitute and see what happens."

Today your standard "I want to free myself" routine seemed to annoy Doctor Simon a tiny bit. Never before had he shown any kind of emotion. You seized this as evidence that he was growing impatient with you.

"Well, why don't you just take off your clothes and do it?" he asked.

But it was so difficult. While you had been coming to this office for almost two years, you still felt as though you were revealing yourself to someone who never shared anything of himself with you. When you said this he came back with, "Come now, you're resisting. We mustn't let the focus of our sessions get blurred. You're here to discuss you, not me."

Today he was softly insistent, urging you on. "There's nothing, nothing at all to fear. I'm here. I'll take care of you."

You felt better. You decided today would really be it. You began to unbutton your blouse. And then your courage left you. But Doctor Simon wouldn't let you back down. He sat next to you on the couch and reassured you.

"Are you afraid I won't think you're pretty?" he asked.

He guided your hand to the next button and the next. Your clothes were slowly coming off. Only your panties and bra were left. You stopped again. You couldn't look him straight in the eye. But he turned your head gently toward him and again reassured you.

"You're lovely, please go on."

You got up and unhooked the bra and let it drop to the carpet. Your large breasts swung free. The nipples hardened as the cool air crossed your body. Doctor Simon couldn't help but stare at your breasts' unexpected size. Usually you wore your clothes one size too large to hide their fullness.

You stepped out of your panties quickly and felt his eyes drop to your silken hair. It too was a surprise, since you were one of those rarities—a natural blonde.

"You are really beautiful, you know," he said softly.

All at once you felt as though you had thrown off the weight of the world. You felt wonderful and started to dance around the room.

"I feel silly," you said, but he encouraged you to act in any way you wished.

"You know, I always wanted to do this as a little girl, but no one in my family ever approved of nudity."

"Well, in here you can be that child again."

You got right into it. You were a kid again. Before you knew it, you were acting playful with Doctor Simon, who seemed pleased—as if playing with his young daughter.

"I want to sit on your lap," you shyly asked. He smiled and nodded approval.

As you sat down and put your arms around his neck, you

couldn't resist the urge to hug him. He gave you a warm hug in return. You embraced for a while and then you thought you detected a reluctance on his part for you to leave his lap. He held you there for a little longer than seemed necessary.

You found yourself unconsciously moving your hands up to his hair and tracing the shape of his face with your fingers.

He held you about the waist very tightly.

"Is . . . is this all right to do?" you stammered, not sure of yourself, but reacting more to an unconscious need.

He didn't answer, nor did he let you go.

Then he seemed to relax. His hand moved upward to caress your bare back very lightly. With his other hand you felt him gently cup your breast. You froze. It was as if, for an instant, you both were sealed in a vacuum. When you didn't stop him, he explored your body further. He kneaded your other breast as you perched very still on his lap. He leaned over and kissed each nipple and began licking and sucking them.

"I . . . I think it will be good for you to practice opening up all your responses," he breathed. "Don't worry, I won't hurt you."

He pushed you slowly down on the couch where you both had been sitting. You were naked and he was completely dressed. "I won't hurt you," he kept whispering.

And since you trusted him more than you trusted any other person in the world, you believed him completely.

Your body was unyielding at first, but it melted as he began kissing your forehead. You just lay there and let him take over. He kissed your eyelids, each cheek, and then your mouth—very gently, until you felt his tongue urge your mouth open. His tongue explored there for a long time. You were so overwhelmed, you felt dizzy and faint.

His lips made their way down your neck to your breasts where he lingered, licking and nibbling at your nipples. As he wended his way on, you took a deep breath and opened your legs to his eager mouth. His hands reached down to cup your buttocks as he raised your wet vagina. He licked the outside first and then, in response to your heavy breathing, he finally darted his tongue inside you. It probed deep into your hot, moist tissue.

Suddenly he raised himself, and you felt his hardness against your leg. You stiffened, afraid.

"I told you not to worry. I won't come in you," he reassured.

He penetrated you, very hot and very hard. And you didn't stop to think that he was dressed and you were naked. You moved your body as hard as you could to match his faster and faster movements. As you were about to come, he pulled himself out and went down to your vagina again and drank and lapped at your juices as you reached your climax.

Later, he readjusted his clothing and helped you to dress. You looked at him in a totally new way. . . .

19

Meeting at the St. Regis

THINKING BACK, YOU should have trusted your instincts. He was just too handsome, too smooth. In short, TROUBLE stood out all over him. But his self-confidence overcame your qualms and you were won over by his charming manner.

He had approached your table in the St. Regis cocktail lounge and smiled. Then he asked if you were alone.

In a few moments he managed to invite himself to join you and he persuaded you to switch from Virgin Marys to Sambuca Romana, a strong, delicious-tasting drink you had never heard of before.

"I'm Italian," he said. "Sambuca is something even my grandfather drank."

After a few more drinks you become aware how deftly he has found out that you're alone, with no plans for that evening. Why, he even has you telling him about some of your lovers!

All this "confession" makes you somewhat uncomfortable and you congratulate yourself on refusing his dinner invitation, explaining that there are some things you really must do at home. While trying to make a graceful exit you let him persuade you to give him your phone number, which he scribbles on a cocktail napkin.

"Call me," you say as you leave.

"I will," he replies, waving the napkin at you.

Whew! You feel like you've escaped a minor ordeal. Yet, you're intrigued. He's fantastic looking. Oh . . . he'll never call.

Surprise! The next evening he has you on the phone and

before you know it, you're on your way to Mona Lisa, a small, family-type Italian restaurant in the Village to meet him for dinner.

Delicious dinner with good red wine, and soon he's telling you how he likes people who are honest with one another. You can't disagree with that. He goes on saying how he could take you to a movie or to dance, but what he'd really like to do is to take you home! You're not running this time and you reach his apartment shortly.

You've never seen anything like it. Particularly the bedroom, where you just about sink to your knees in carpeting as you enter.

He has continued pouring red wine while giving you the tour of his apartment. In a few moments the two of you are locked together on the llama rug barely able to get out of your clothing before making love violently, quickly, and falling asleep in each other's arms.

As you awaken later your head feels so foggy. It takes you a few moments to figure out the strange feeling you're having. You look around to see your hands and legs bound to each of the four posts of the bed. And as you look up, he's standing right above you with his penis hanging down.

"What?. . ." you begin to say.

"Shut up," he says pleasantly. "You're my prisoner."

You don't know why, but you're not afraid. You decide it's a game and you'll go along with it. He couldn't really be planning to hurt you—not with that warm smile. As if in answer to your unspoken question, he leans down and kisses you. In a swift motion, he forces his penis into your mouth. In another motion he takes his penis down to your cunt and whips it against you.

"This is cunt whipping," he explains.

He does this for a while and it gets you quite aroused. Afterwards he moves back to your face and tells you to lick his balls. As you do you watch him in fascination while he pulls his penis roughly. You hear his breathing become husky and he moves away enough to enable him to come—all over your face. It squirts all over and where it doesn't reach, he rubs it into you with his hands.

Once again he demands that you lick his balls. You take them into your mouth and suck on them as he gets hard again. The scene is repeated but this time he comes all over your breasts.

You don't even believe it's possible that within a few more minutes he's erect again and now he's fucking you. You can't really move since he's got you tied. You can only receive what he offers.

After fucking you for a while, he leaves the bed, only to return quickly with the robe belt from his bathrobe. He starts gently whipping you across your body. And then he stands over you. You can't even imagine what he'll do next. You feel warm liquid dripping on you and you realize he's urinating! When he's finished he turns around with his buttocks in your face.

"Lick my asshole," he demands.

When you hesitate, he whips your cunt with the belt—only this time, it hurts a bit. And so you stick your tongue into his asshole. You lick and probe and you feel his penis getting hard again as it presses against your breasts. He has you keep this up for a long time as he jerks off against you and comes one more time before falling asleep on top of you.

Much later he unties your hands and feet and acts as if nothing unusual has happened. He's the charming guy you met at the cocktail lounge.

He helps you to shower and even towels you dry. You decline sleeping there, but he makes sure to put you into a cab so that you'll get home—safely.

Author's note: Among those who helped shape my manuscript into a finished book were many women who questioned the inclusion of the fantasy you've just read. Most admitted that it excited them. But they also objected that they "just didn't like it." Balancing the pros and cons, I hewed to my original purpose which was, after all, to challenge and excite. Thus it remains.

20

The Delivery Boy

SINCE JOHN DIED seven months ago, life had become a mechanical passing of time. Nothing was important anymore; you had nothing left to do. But the hours had to be filled. How had twenty-one years passed so quickly? Only when there is a loss does one become aware of how interdependent a husband and wife can be.

Friends tried—and continued to try—to help occupy you. But it all ended by being alone once more . . . no matter how many weekends spent at a sister-in-law's home, no matter how many hours passed at concerts, films . . .

What no one had prepared you for was the physical loss. You found yourself desperate for love. You had no idea how to satisfy this gnawing need. Women of your age had been brought up to think of "touching themselves" as dirty. You weren't sure what you were supposed to do, even if you had the nerve to try.

That morning the same as every day—you'd read the *Times* from the front-page headlines to the television listings—drank another cup of coffee—anything for a semblance of activity and purpose. The doorbell startled you. Who could that be? But when the voice informed you that the package from the department store had arrived, you recalled the shopping trip a week ago.

As you opened the door a wave of heat almost knocked you down as it rushed into the cool, air-conditioned apartment. The poor fellow stood there, practically drenched in perspiration, holding the package in his hand.

You were signing the receipt when he cleared his throat. "I beg your pardon, but could I bother you for a glass of water?"

You felt almost embarrassed by your hesitation. He hardly seemed the threatening type. But you learn to live by certain rules, and one is *never* to let a strange man into one's home.

"Forget it, lady," he said, both angry and frustrated.

"No, no, please come in," you replied, somehow concerned about hurting this young man's feelings. "It's just that. . ."

"I know, I know," he answered with a sigh. "Everyone is so suspicious these days. But it's really roasting out there. I really *would* appreciate a drink of water."

You both stood there awkwardly for another moment. But finally a friendly smile passed between you. You stepped aside to allow him in the apartment.

"This is great. It's really cool in here," he sighed. "Sure beats riding around in a delivery truck all day."

As you showed him into the kitchen, you became aware of your flimsy clothing. You wore only a robe over your sheer nightgown. What thoughts you were having! For heaven's sake. Here was a fellow not much older than your own son and you were concerned that he'd even notice what you were wearing.

You handed him the drink and saw him suddenly flush. His eyes avoided yours. Why? Had he been watching you? You didn't have a bad figure for a woman your age. Actually you had a pretty good figure for a woman of any age. You'd seen many young girls who would spend years dieting and exercising and *never* look the way you did. All that tennis and swimming had paid off.

You found yourself trying to engage him in conversation: "Have you worked for this company very long?

"Do they treat you well?

"Do you go to school?"

He seemed in no rush to leave and it wasn't long before you knew that his name was Larry, and he was planning to go to law school at night while holding down this job during the day.

"You know," he suddenly said, "you're about the nicest person I've met since I've worked on this job. I guess I really should go now, though."

This was more of a question than a statement and you urged him to stay a while longer.

"I have nothing to do today, so you don't have to hurry on my account. Actually," you explained, "since my husband died, I seem to have nothing *but* free time."

You couldn't help it. You were feeling sorry for yourself again. The tears started. You were quite sure Larry was embarrassed, but instead of running away he came over to you and placed his hand on your shoulder. "Please don't cry," he implored gently.

You reached up to touch his hand. He didn't draw away. For a long moment neither of you said anything.

"I know you must be very lonely," Larry said, "but you should get out and meet people. You're terrific looking. I'll bet you attract lots of men."

The flattery was just what you needed. When his hand moved toward the opening of your robe, it seemed to be the most natural thing to happen. He looked at you directly without averting his eyes. "Most girls *my* age don't look half as lovely," he continued.

What a smooth talker he was. Even though you knew it was foolish, you didn't care. You wanted to hear tender words, and Larry sensed this.

"Come here," he said and offered you his hand. You followed him like a child to the couch in the living room. He sat down, pulling you next to him and took your face in both of his hands kissing you lightly on the mouth. Your mouth eagerly returned his kisses, which grew more and more passionate.

He took your robe off and fondled your body through the

tricot of your nightgown. As he began to remove that too, you froze for an instant. What were you doing? He was a boy! It was ridiculous. But when you heard him breathing so heavily, you realized he wasn't responding like a boy. He lay on top of you, the fabric of his uniform rough against the softness of your gown. You felt his hardness rising as he kissed and stroked you.

When you parted briefly, he gently pulled the gown over your head. You were unsure of yourself again, but saw only pleasure in his eyes. "You're beautiful," he breathed. This was no line now. He seemed truly startled and he quickly took off his jacket and shirt, revealing a firm, hairless, chest. He drew you to him and his body felt wonderful against yours. You could have stayed in that embrace for hours. But he soon drew away to quickly remove the rest of his clothing. You were both naked, facing each other.

You looked at his young, firm body and opened your arms to him. He came eagerly, already hard. He inserted himself inside you slowly, as if afraid he might hurt you.

How long had it been since there had been a man between your legs? You hungrily began moving against him. You urged him on—you wanted to feel his strength deep inside you. It felt so wonderful. You could hear yourself saying, "It's so good, so wonderful, so good, so good . . ."

He kissed you harder now and forced his tongue into your mouth. You sucked on it, tasting its moisture. He kept moving to and fro even while he explored the rest of your body, rubbing your nipples and kissing your throat as he groaned, moving closer and closer to climax. You were terribly excited by his sounds and your body moved automatically in a rhythm totally attuned to his. He moved his hand to play with your clitoris. Your head started pounding, there was a dryness in your throat. You could hardly keep from swallowing Larry up—you clung to him so closely.

He encircled your clitoris with his fingers as it stood out hard, all while he continued moving in you. Your legs went rigid; your buttocks tightened almost painfully. It was upon you so quickly that your body shook with the power of the climax. Larry let go then and with one more thrust, he let his seed rush into you. He kept pumping afterwards as if trying to pour every drop he had into your receptive body.

You lay there for a long time, all of you still pulsating as he cradled you in his arms.

Later, after he'd gone you remained contentedly prone on the sofa and thought of how he hadn't said goodbye. He just left quietly.

You didn't know if you'd ever see Larry again. But that didn't seem to be the most important thing. All that mattered was the wonderful feeling that filled you at that moment.

21

The Sisters

YOU HAD JUST slipped into your nightgown when the door to your bedroom opened, startling you. In the doorway stood Mel, a friend of your dad's who was staying the night.

What a weird coincidence! That very moment you had been daydreaming about him! He was about your father's age—forty-five or so—but he seemed much younger. He dressed like a guy half his age, wore his hair long, and sported a very sexy beard and mustache. You always figured he hardly knew you existed. After all, you were only sixteen—a kid—and you had kept your crush on him to yourself all these months he had been visiting your home.

But here he was, standing in his pajamas, just staring at you.

"Say," he muttered, trying to find an excuse for being there, "do you have anything to read? I can't fall asleep without reading something in bed."

"Sure, I'll find something." You were surprised at how calm you sounded, even though your heart was pounding and you felt the flush on your cheeks. "Come on in and shut the door," you added, trying to be casual.

Mel didn't need much encouragement. He sat himself on the edge of your bed while you plopped down next to him, going through some magazines. Impulsively you turned toward him and untied the rope of his pajama bottoms, which fell open, exposing a rigid penis. He sat there frozen. You reached for him and began to massage it as it got firmer. He sighed and lay back on the bed passively as you continued.

You wondered if he was thinking how childish you looked. You had your hair in braids and wore a baby-doll nightgown, making you look even younger than your age. Well, whatever he thought, he certainly was not resisting your caresses.

You leaned down and took him in your mouth. You sucked expertly, making his body move in time with your tongue and grasping mouth. You moved your hands underneath his buttocks and caressed his balls, while continuing to suck up and down. He began to moan softly and move more violently.

Just then you heard the door opening, and you both were motionless. It was Julia, your older sister. She obviously had been peeking through the keyhole and was very turned on by the scene. She still had her hand between her legs as she entered.

"Don't stop," she whispered. "I'll just join you, if you don't mind."

Neither of you responded, so Julia sat on the bed, at a distance, and continued to play with herself. You both stopped to watch her when she had brought herself almost to the point of orgasm, but she stopped until she cooled off a bit. After she had teased herself this way several times, she leaned closer to Mel and you, wanting to join in.

Julia and you turned your attention to Mel, stroking his chest and balls and taking turns sucking on his throbbing cock. Almost unconsciously Julia reached for you and began fondling your budding breasts. You accepted this as if it were a common occurrence and responded by touching her. In a few minutes you were playing with each other fervently, exciting each other as much as you were exciting Mel, who lay between you.

From his movements, it was clear that Mel was ready to burst. Just then he pulled his cock out of your mouth and pushed both Julia's and your face close together, at the level of his hot rod. He came—squirting all over you. This got you so excited that you began to come at the same time while Julia returned her hand to between her legs and quickly brought herself off as well.

"The Browner The Berry . . ."

THERE WAS SOMETHING exotic about Grace. People were always surprised when they noticed her eyes were light green. Since not many people had ever seen a black person with light eyes, there was usually speculation over the "purity" of her blackness. It made her very unusual.

Not that the rest of her was commonplace — her hair was worn in the latest style and it framed her smooth dark face. Her features were broad and aggressive and always looked challenging. She had the body of an athlete and, indeed, played tennis often and thus kept herself firm. Her ass was special, too — jutting out like a shelf behind her. You always wanted to reach out and touch it.

You often wondered what attracted her to you. You were fairly pretty, but almost the complete opposite of Grace. Your skin was a honey color, and your overall appearance was softer. You probably gravitated toward one another because of the anger you shared over the lack of interesting black men in this small town and the arrogant attitude that many of the white men still had toward black girls — that they could take them without worrying about the consequences.

At first you and Grace had merely met and griped about it all. But one night when you had gotten mellow, you let it all hang out.

She stood up in her aggressive way and asked — to no one in particular — why nobody appreciated her value. She had impulsively stripped bare as if to demonstrate her worth. As she pranced around, all the time stroking her beautiful breasts and running her hands over her big ass, she had aired her complaints. At first you were amused, but being rather high yourself, you followed her lead and stripped also, to show your own body.

Soon your high was gone and you found yourself depressed and in tears at the injustice of it all. Grace came over to comfort you and brush your tears away. She held you in an almost motherly way as she stroked your back. You put your arms around her, and, like opposite poles of a magnet, your mouths were suddenly drawn together. You were greedily kissing and tasting each other's tongues.

This led quite naturally to the rest.

Grace took the lead. Her hungry full mouth moved over you. You thought vaguely of the different color tones of your bodies blending while twisting about on your bed. You felt that this was what you had been missing. There was no guilt—men were not involved at all.

You reached for that delightful ass and held onto it while you buried your mouth into her bush. You felt the drops of moisture and your tongue greedily sought out the honey. Grace's hands moved without stopping. She brushed the downy fuzz at the small of your back as you sighed. She began to massage your buttocks and probed gently around your anus with her finger. She worked it around the tight rim at first and then slowly inserted it. You loved it and moved so that she could massage you better. Now you were lying on your stomach and she was above you, fucking you with her finger.

She paused only for a moment and then you felt her replace her finger with something larger. It was a candle which she pushed slowly in and out. At the same time she reached around and massaged your clitoris. No man had ever done this. You closed your eyes and pictured what was happening.

As she continued her rubbing, you heard yourself shouting, "I'm going to come. . . ."

As you did, she moved her mouth down to drink all your juices and kept licking and massaging and moving the candle until you thought you would faint.

As soon as you had recovered, she moved quickly and silently so that her black wiry muff was directly over your face. Automatically your tongue reached out for it, and she squealed with delight as she began to grind her pussy onto your eager mouth.

She looked fabulous from that view. Her black breasts hovered over your face for you to stroke and slap playfully. It didn't take very long for her grinding motions to quicken and then she said, "That's it, yes, yes, that's it," and you knew you had the spot. You wanted to tease her, but her body was insistent and she bore down hard on your mouth.

Soon she uttered a cry that was more animal than human. As she came, she started jerking up and down for a long time. When she had fallen off you, you both fell into a deep, contented sleep.

23

The Schoolgirls

YOU WERE PRAYING they wouldn't call your mother. Gosh! If she found out, she'd really beat you. How could you and Flo have let yourselves get caught that way?

You hadn't heard a thing until the teacher's horrified scream. "My God, what are you girls doing?"

Now you were sure to get kicked out of this boarding school, too. You already could hear your mother saying, "What will we do with her now? She's only thirteen. . . ."

Now you were being brought to the dean's office, and both you and Flo were terrified at what he'd do to you.

After you were seated in front of Dean Kenton, he assured the teacher he could handle the situation. She left and the three of you were face to face. You and Flo waited.

Dean Kenton began rather sternly, "Girls, Miss Coleman tells me she discovered you in the locker room doing some sort of physical thing to each other." He shriveled you with his stare.

"Do you know exactly what it means, what you were doing?"

Neither of you could find your tongue. "Well, surely you know that we can't have girls behaving in a way that will upset the entire school," he continued. "But as a policy I want to be fair so I never reprimand my students for actions I have not myself witnessed. Now if you want to deny that you were doing anything, I will turn the matter over to the school board."

You sat, frozen with fright.

"There's another possibility," he continued. "If you show me exactly what you were doing, I will be able to judge for myself and perhaps handle the whole thing just in this room."

You sat silently, not quite understanding what he expected of you until he repeated himself.

"Well girls, will you please demonstrate *exactly* what you were doing to each other when you were, er, apprehended."

Still you sat. But he got firmer and began to sound angry. "Stand up!"

You both did.

"Were you undressed?" he asked.

"Yes," you managed to whisper.

"Well then, let's get on with it."

You exchanged glances with Flo before beginning to shyly undress, right there in front of him.

Soon you were down to panties and bras. Flo was your age and your girlish figures were just starting to turn into those of young women. You each had budding little breasts and the beginning of hair between your legs.

"Now," Dean Kenton frowned, "this is not being totally undressed." So you removed the last fragile garments.

"Now why don't you go over to that couch and show me what you were up to," he directed.

You moved hesitantly to the couch and slowly lay down next to each other.

"Go on, go on," he said impatiently, from his desk across the room.

You turned so your head was facing her little slit and hers was close to yours. You opened her legs and she did the same to you. Then you glanced over to Dean Kenton, who still looked very somber.

"Please continue," was all he said.

You began to lick her where you had before, and she automatically returned your caresses with her tongue. You had been doing this for several months after discovering each other one evening in the dormitory, and you got together as often as you could. You thought of her all day long in class. Flo also found it hard to concentrate on square roots and Washington crossing the Delaware.

Now in front of Dean Kenton, you were scared and shy, but it still felt so good that your legs relaxed in moments and opened as wide as you could make them to let Flo reach as much of you as possible. You got into it, too, enthusiastically licking at her delicious body. She had even less hair than you, and there was nothing to interfere with your probing tongue.

You heard Dean Kenton's chair slide against the floor as he rose and walked slowly toward you. "Don't stop, girls," he said, "I want to see it all."

You didn't want to stop, it was too sweet. Very soon you were coming and, carried along with your excitement, Flo quickly reached her own climax. You let up a bit but Dean Kenton didn't seem satisfied.

"I think you'd best do it again. I want to be sure I haven't missed anything," he said.

You could feel the heat from Dean Kenton's body as you repeated your game. He pushed his face very close as you licked at Flo, almost as if he were trying to peer right inside her. Then he moved to where she was licking.

For all of your experimentation, you were really quite innocent. Flo and you only knew that what you were doing felt so great, you wanted to do it as often as possible. But that was all it meant.

Your tongue was beginning to ache when Dean Kenton finally told you to stop. You stood there dripping and naked before him.

"Well, I suppose you know I must punish the both of you, don't you?"

You nodded and waited for his decision. "Well, I'm going

to spank you very hard so you won't forget your punishment. You first," he said, and turned you over his knee.

He held you very tightly to him. "So you won't slip off," he said, and you felt something beneath you, poking into your stomach, very hard. "Now don't move and don't cry out, or I'll have to do it all over again," he instructed.

And then he beckoned to Flo and told her that she must stand over you so that you would be sure not to move. When she was in the proper position, her little breasts were very close to Dean Kenton's face.

He began to spank you. He said he would rub your backside each time so that it wouldn't hurt as much. He would spank and then make a very large circle with his hand and sort of press downward, right to where you felt that poking from underneath. He did this slowly for a while, and then he started to spank faster and harder. All the time Flo leaned down over you so you wouldn't move.

After several minutes you turned your head a bit and saw he was very red in the face. You guessed that he must have been angrier than he admitted. You were going to have to bear it until it was over.

He kept spanking harder and faster, and you started to cry because it really hurt. And then suddenly he gave you one good, hard spank and that was the end. The poking seemed to stop, too, and you were glad to have it finished.

Flo was very upset, knowing what was in store for her. She was staring fearfully at your bright red buttocks. But Dean Kenton surprised you by saying, "Well, Flo, I think we'll put off your punishment until tomorrow. I don't want to make it too hard on you girls. After all, I know you didn't mean any harm."

He seemed to smile slightly as he told you, "Now report back to me tomorrow, both of you, and we'll finish this off."

24

Seducing the Masseuse

IT WAS A long train ride but you were so wrapped up with the idea of meeting Artie again, you hardly paid the least bit of attention to the time. You'd been apart for several weeks, and you were terribly horny. Masturbating had given you relief, but your body ached for the contact of him against you. You could almost feel him inside you. Whenever you thought about it, your legs trembled and your juices started to flow.

Artie met you at the station. After a long hello kiss, he held you very close to him and said, "I've got a surprise for you. In two hours you are going to have a massage in the privacy of our motel room."

You guess you looked disappointed. You'd been looking forward to spending several hours alone together, and now he was supplying you with a masseuse instead.

But he reassured you. "It'll set you up beautifully for a long session in bed. You'll see. She's a lovely girl, and I think I can talk her into giving you a sensual massage."

Your first reaction was negative, but as you rode towards the motel, your mind wandered. You always loved being massaged, and it was one of your fantasies that the masseuse would let her fingers slip. . . . Hmmm, the thought alone excited you.

You unpacked and had a light lunch in the dining room. A few minutes after you got back to the room, the masseuse arrived. She was a young girl, not more than twenty-four, tall, and even through her uniform you could see her pointy breasts pushing against the fabric. She was very "officially" dressed. White dress, white stockings, and white shoes.

Artie said, "You massage her first and then me."

"All right," the masseuse replied and gave him a shy smile. You gathered they'd talked beforehand about a sensual massage, but she gave no indication that she'd give one.

You undressed quickly and felt chilled. The room was cold. The girl led you to a portable massage table which she had brought along. As you lay down, she covered you with a sheet. Artie lowered the lights, "to set the mood," he explained with a hint of a laugh.

She began to massage you as you lay face up. Her hands were strong and forceful. She started with your face, and you relaxed completely—the dim lighting helping to further the feeling of intimacy. Your eyes closed and your mind wandered. You didn't particularly care if the massage was sensual or not because your body responded sensually to any kind of touch.

As she moved her hands down to your arms and chest, you heard a rustling sound and realized that Artie was trying to persuade her to really work over your breasts.

"No, please," she said, in a low pleading whisper. "I can't do it. I wish I could, but I'm too nervous. I've never given anything other than a straight massage. If they found out, I'd lose my job here."

"Well, just massage her breasts," Artie said.

She must have agreed to this because you felt her fingers move in circles around them until finally she touched your nipples. At first she barely brushed them, as if afraid she'd be struck by a bolt of lightning. Then she became braver. She kneaded your breasts gently but very firmly. Her focus changed soon and she moved down your body. As she massaged the inside of your thighs, you could almost swear she let her hand brush past your pubic hair. (Perhaps it was your overactive imagination. . . .) Your body was squirming with responsiveness—especially since it had been so long since you'd been stroked by someone.

You could sense Artie trying to urge her further, and every so often she begged off, saying how uncomfortable she felt.

She asked if we had any grass because she thought that it might loosen her up if she smoked a little. We didn't. You felt her discomfort and asked Artie not to continue to force her.

When the massage ended, you felt wonderfully relaxed.

Next it was Artie's turn. He disrobed and got up on the table. She began to massage him and as she did, you couldn't contain your need to touch him. You moved around to the foot of the table and began to run your hands along his legs. When you drew near to his penis it began to stiffen. You looked at the girl and she smiled, indicating that she didn't mind your presence, so you continued. You fondled his penis and were about to take it in your mouth. Before you could, Artie spoke up to the masseuse. "Have you ever had a massage yourself?"

"Oh, no," she said. "Who would give me one? My husband doesn't—"

"Why don't you let us? I'll bet you'd enjoy it."

Her cheeks began to color and she started to decline when Artie slipped off the table and holding her hand, gently pulled her toward it.

"Come on," he said. "Just for a few minutes."

"You'll enjoy it," you said encouragingly. "Why don't you just relax?"

You seemed to give her the reassurance she needed because she took her clothes off. Everything but her panties. She lay on the table and you pulled them down with both hands. She didn't resist.

She really had a voluptuous body. Her breasts were firm and big and had very large nipples. They'd been concealed by her loose dress. She had a tiny waist which accentuated her rather full hips. Her stomach was completely flat as she lay on her back and only her jutting hipbones interrupted the smooth line from one side to the other. Her hair was dark and plentiful and her legs, though slightly heavy, didn't have an ounce of flab. She had a fading scar, apparently from a Caesarean birth. Somehow it made her more attractive. . . .

Artie and you began your amateur massage. After a little while she did relax—trusting you now—and really began to enjoy it. You moved your hands up to her breasts and began to knead them as she had yours. Artie was now running his palms down her legs, letting his fingertips brush her pubic hair. Her eyes closed and her mouth slackened involuntarily. She was obviously responding to your manipulations.

You changed places with Artie and became more aggressive with your fingers as you let them slip along the outside of the lips of her vagina. Her legs opened as you stroked her. All resistance was gone. Artie gestured silently to you and you both began to suck on her nipples which hardened quickly. You kept lightly playing inside her with your fingers. She was wet now and her legs parted even more as you rubbed expertly at the soft folds of her cunt.

The move from massage table to bed was swift, and the three of you fell into a dreamlike love-making that was totally natural and automatic—as if you'd known each other all your lives.

She reached hungrily for your breasts and began to suck at them as greedily as a baby needing milk. You continued fondling her body and then took your place at her breasts, licking them avidly. Artie spread apart the outer folds of her vagina and buried his face between her legs. She loved this and began to coo and murmur almost inaudibly how wonderful it felt. At the same time she reached up for your face and you kissed for a long time. You moved to straddle her face, putting your bush at her mouth.

She took to this immediately and lapped at you as if trying

to capture every bit of juice that oozed out of your burning body. You kept lowering and raising yourself, and she followed you with her tongue until you started to come. You didn't want to finish that quickly, so, reluctantly, you climbed down.

As you did, Artie left her for a moment and went behind you. He plunged his hard cock into you with no prelude, no foreplay. Oh! You'd been wanting that after the long weeks of separation. How marvelous it felt as you moved together. You began to lap at her moist slit which lay beneath you, and you continued to pleasure her. You don't know how long it went on like this.

Eventually, Artie pulled out of you and again went down on her as you moved away. She was close to coming and you watched her as she got closer and closer. Her face was contorted with frustration as she seemed unable to lose herself completely. You kept playing with her nipples and running your hands over her body as she moved closer to her climax.

Without warning you climbed back up to her hungry mouth, and she ate you again. As her tongue flicked across your clit, she went off violently. Her sucking and nibbling pushed you into that same erupting volcano.

You smiled at each other warmly and embraced one another as if in gratitude for the pleasure you had exchanged.

You drew apart finally and both of you turned to Artie who had given so unselfishly all this time. Now it was his turn.

25

The Last Taboo

FOR A LONG time you've had a very strong physical attraction for Daddy. Tonight it's just Daddy and you. You're alone because your mother has gone to the country to visit relatives. It's late in the evening and the television, turned very low, is making a soft, bubbling sound in the background.

"Hey, Dad," you say, "I have some questions for you."

"What about?" he asks.

You walk over and stand above him. You know that your breasts are clearly visible through your very sheer blouse. You lean over and kiss him on the forehead, deliberately making sure that a breast is close to his face.

His hand falls from your shoulder down to your waist, but on the way it touches a nipple and you feel an instant thrill—although you're fairly certain it was accidental.

"Dad, what are we going to do this weekend?"

"Haven't given it much thought."

You swing around and sit on his lap the way you did when you were a little girl. He puts his arm around you, but now you're no longer that flat-chested child. He has his hand very close to one of your breasts, not for any purpose it would seem, just casually placed there.

As you're perched on one of his knees, you start absently rubbing your thigh, knowing full well that the back of your hand is rubbing near his penis. At first there's no reaction. In a few moments, though, you feel a beginning hardness. You look into his eyes innocently. Both of you act as though nothing is happening and both of you pretend to carry on some sort of conversation.

As if perfectly matter of factly, you guide his fingers to your right breast. Then you kiss him on the lips. He stands up. Nothing more is said. He picks you up and carries you into your bedroom.

"Are you putting me to sleep, Daddy?" you ask as he lays you down, but your voice isn't natural.

"Kind of," he answers. He now has his hand between your legs, and he moves it up, brushing your scant pubic hair and stroking your vagina. You're so wet you're almost ashamed.

"Oh, Daddy."

Your father looks at you, then lifts your head up and kisses you on the cheek, on the forehead, and on the lips. You reach over and unzip his fly. Almost before you know it, his pants are off and his firm cock is over you. He spreads your legs and slowly but steadily inserts himself into you. You close your eyes and think how wonderful it feels.

"Oh, Daddy, oh Daddy, I love you," you say.

"And I love you," he says.

26

A Girl's Best Friend

TODAY IS LIKE any other day. You're about to make yourself some coffee when the doorbell rings. You open it, and there's your girl friend Sheila. She's brought a big-boned silver German shepherd with her. You hadn't realized she owned a dog. They come in, and you offer her a cup of coffee.

Ignoring your question, and barely able to contain herself, she blurts out, "How would you like to see what I've trained Rex to do?" You're not sure what she means, but you agree to watch. "Wait till you see," she says. "Rex is a very special dog."

She suggests going into the bedroom. You follow her, more puzzled than ever. She lies down on your bed, pulls off her panties, and arranges her skirt so that her cunt is bared. As if on cue, the dog goes to her and sniffs around her. He licks around her stomach and her ass as if smelling his way to familiar territory. Then at last he licks at her labia and she sighs audibly. As his reddish tongue moves across her pudendum, she spreads her legs wider. She begins to squirm as Rex laps away, occasionally forcing his large tongue into her vagina.

It's an astonishing sight and you feel yourself becoming excited, too. You can't take your eyes off the scene, where Rex's tongue never pauses. Your hand unconsciously reaches down between your own legs and you start playing on top of your panties. When you become aware of what you're doing, you're a little startled, but you see that Sheila is in her own private world. So you reach down into your panties and begin to caress yourself more openly.

After the dog licks Sheila for a few more minutes, she begins to moan. Her face contorts as her body makes itself ready for a tremendous release. You take your hand away from your snatch and watch, fascinated as she emits a low, animal-like sound while she climaxes.

When her composure returns, she adjusts her-clothing and asks if you'd like Rex to perform his carnal trick on you. Your immediate answer is, "No, I couldn't—" Your flushed face gives you away. She knows you're lying. Gently she urges you on, telling you how much you'll enjoy it, insisting she'd get a great deal of pleasure watching Rex going down on you.

It doesn't take much prodding before you lie down on the bed and spread your legs. The dog moves right in, sniffing away, as he did to Sheila. He's inquisitive at first, licking your stomach, then your ass, and finally your cunt which is juicing heavily from your own foreplay while watching Sheila.

The dog's enthusiasm has diminished, though, and you're becoming very frustrated. Sheila has an idea. She goes into the kitchen and brings out some raw hamburger. She has you lie back down. She rubs some of the meat on the lips of your cunt. The dog becomes quite aroused and licks at you with new fervor. She keeps replacing the meat as the dog's gravelly tongue wipes it away.

Your eyes close while your body reacts automatically. Your hips move and you let out muffled sounds of delight. You love it.

You feel yourself getting close to orgasm, but Rex takes his head away again. "Don't stop!" you groan. Sheila, seeing that you're so close to getting off, tries to hold the dog close to your cunt. He refuses to lick any more. Fully aware of your rising frustration, Sheila quickly replaces the dog and runs her own tongue along your clit, in and out of your cunt and within moments, you do come. It's so lovely you don't move. You just smile at your friend and then take her in your arms and kiss her as she lies quietly next to you.

A Group Meeting With The Internist

WHEN DOCTOR LANG called you to tell you he had a group of women who were interested in talking over some of the sex problems they shared, you said at once that you would be willing to join.

Now, on your way to his office, you began to wonder why an internist was so concerned about the emotional problems of his patients. In a way, it impressed you to think he was willing to become involved to this extent in a day when most doctors were rather impersonal.

But as you thought about it, it occurred to you that Doctor Lang had always seemed different. Almost from the start he had asked questions that no other physician ever asked. Like, "Do you fantasize?" Or, "Have you ever considered having sex with someone other than your husband?"

"What are your thoughts about group sex?" And so on.

At first you had been startled by these questions, but he reassured you, explaining that he was interested in the emotional as well as the physical well-being of his patients, since they were, in his opinion, interrelated. And of course, this was all very confidential. And . . . well . . . actually, you found that it titillated you a bit. You always left his office with your cheeks burning up, feeling very high.

The last visit followed pretty much the same routine. This time, when his nurse left the examining room for a moment, he said something about running an experiment which might help women who had trouble reaching orgasm.

It was a matter-of-fact comment, and he didn't dwell on it. But it stayed in your mind. Especially since your sex life with Ralph had become rather humdrum, and you were climaxing less often these days, as if you'd both lost the touch. In fact, you couldn't remember the last time you had an orgasm!

But you were still surprised at your quick, positive response when Doctor Lang told you about the group. Despite your ambivalence, you were determined to attend. You were also curious to see some of his other patients and to find out what kind of sex problems they had.

You didn't run into much traffic on your way over, and as you parked the car, you wondered why you hadn't told Ralph where you were going. Were you afraid he wouldn't approve? Well, no, you just thought he wouldn't understand, so what was the point?

Your finger hovered over the doorbell. There was still time to change your mind. Too late you thought to yourself as your finger moved forward to press it.

Doctor Lang greeted you warmly. He wasn't in his white examining jacket, and he looked different and very handsome. As a matter of fact, you didn't recall ever seeing him out of "uniform" before. He quickly ushered you into his consulting room where there were three other women. They were very much like yourself, you concluded. Young, in their early thirties, all could benefit from the loss of a few pounds, but, you noted, a bit jealously, that one of them was outstandingly good looking.

Each of you were stealing looks at the others. And you all seemed just a bit uncomfortable.

"Please relax," Doctor Lang said. "We're all here to exchange views and perhaps help one another."

He began to give some sort of explanation of what procedure we would follow and you found yourself not paying much attention until you heard, ". . . should really be kept sort of confidential, between members of this group."

No one protested or questioned. . . . Eventually you were almost at ease, no doubt helped by the sherry he served, and soon were talking quite openly. Marriage wasn't as fulfilling any more. Your husbands were always busy thinking of other things, worried about bosses, deals, recession, inflation. You all felt young and sexy, and there seemed no way to revive interest at home.

"Well," Doctor Lang interrupted, "I think I may be able to help. I'm going to suggest some exercises for you to do alone and with each other which you will eventually teach your husbands."

We were all eager to learn.

"I think the best way to get to know your bodies is to undress," he said.

After an uneasy murmur, he quickly added, "Now, you all have been examined a number of times by me, so you needn't be embarrassed." When no one made a move or a sound, he added, "I'll tell you what, although this is unusual, if it will make you more comfortable, I will also undress so you won't feel I'm merely standing there, not participating. . . .

Before I could make up my mind about the logic of his remark, Doctor Lang had removed his jacket and tie. Then he went over to the tall redhead and helped remove her dress—just like that, while we all watched. (I cursed myself for not having started that reducing diet!)

"Now," he said, "let's all follow through."

He said it with such authority that we did just that. When we had all undressed, we sat naked, with Doctor Lang, in a circle.

"Now I want one of you to lie in the middle." No one moved so he reached out and pulled *me* gently to the center.

"First you should explore your own bodies," he said, and he took my hand to demonstrate. He moved it slowly down my body, pausing at each breast. He applied his own hand for pressure. He had me play with both my nipples. And then his hand and mine continued downward, rubbing a circle on my stomach, and then further down to my triangle of black hair.

Just then he asked another of the women to join us.

"I want to show you how to pleasure yourselves and each other as well." He was speaking softly.

He directed me to spread my legs so that my labia were completely in view. He gently parted the lips. I would have rather been caught shoplifting at the neighborhood deli than lying there. Still, I had a feeling of pleasure and excitement, too.

He called the others around in front of me and said, "I want you to watch as I show her one way to masturbate."

We were all silent and, I'm sure, too shocked to protest. And yet, as I looked quickly at the other women, I saw their eyes as bright and as excited as I knew mine appeared to them. We seemed programmed to follow Doctor Lang's orders.

"Now place your hands on either side of her vagina and open her legs wide."

Two of them did this and I, following his instructions, began to rub my clitoris with my finger. Next I investigated the inside of my vagina, until he instructed each of the others to touch me as well. At first they were reluctant, but then more courageous, and before long I felt myself reaching the point where I knew I was going to climax.

Doctor Lang interrupted my upward arc to say, "I will show you how your husbands can help you maintain your level of excitement and also aid you in achieving orgasm."

Telling me to continue my massage, he placed himself in front of me, between my legs. First he guided my fingers with his. Then he removed my hand and replaced it with his own, in perfect imitation of my motions.

"You see," he whispered, "your husbands can learn to massage you exactly as you do it to yourselves." He manipulated my clitoris as I had. Again I felt that orgasm mounting.

"And now," his voice was lower, soothing, gentle, "I will insert my penis and continue to massage the clitoris without disturbing the flow of feeling."

I was so carried away by now that he could have inserted anything he wanted into me. I felt two things that quickly melted into one uninterrupted motion. He kept up the gentle pressure on my clitoris, but with the other hand he had opened my vagina and implanted his penis into it. He was quite hard and slipped in easily. My body rose to meet his gentle thrust. He proceeded, timing his manual massage perfectly with his penis.

"Keep in time with me," he whispered hoarsely, very close to my ear. I followed his instructions, completely entranced, with absolutely no will of my own.

The others just sat and watched, eyes fixed on the two of us. We moved in tandem until he brought me to a wonderful climax. He kept up his movements as I came and then as I subsided, he gently withdrew.

He hadn't come, I thought, all of that was really just for me. . . .

As I rejoined the group after this delicious interlude, he turned to the woman next to me and drew her into the center of the circle.

And so it went until everyone had been "instructed." We all agreed that a weekly seminar would certainly be a worthwhile undertaking.

29

White Man, Black Man and White Girl

AS YOU ENTERED Vic's hotel room, there was tension between you and Dan. You had made no secret about your brief affair with Vic the last time he'd been in town. Dan had even seemed to approve of it. After all, he pointed out, he had been away at the time, and he didn't believe in fidelity for its own sake—especially if no one was being hurt. Dan admitted, however, that he was surprised to have found himself responding jealously when you told him. He asked you not to screw Vic again.

You dropped the matter and so did Vic. Neither of you felt your "affair" was a love match but rather, a kind of natural, extension of your three-way friendship. Still, you always wondered if part of Dan's jealousy wasn't because Vic was black and because in your openness in describing the love-making, you more or less confirmed the myth, at least in this case, about black men.

You remember being astonished at the size of Vic's cock. And when Dan innocently questioned you about it; you blurted out that it was the biggest you'd ever seen. And Vic knew how to use it as well.

But that was a year ago. Vic had returned to France, and you had gone about your lives. Letters were exchanged and then came the news that he'd be in town again to do a photo layout for his magazine. Now you were all meeting for a drink.

When Vic opened the door to his room, he embraced you both warmly and only you could tell from the turned-down corners of Dan's mouth that this was a difficult reunion for him. You made small talk, but eventually ran out of things to say. You were startled when Dan asked, "Do you remember that last time you were in town? You two got it on together, right?"

Vic and you exchanged looks. You realized he didn't know how to respond, so you quickly said, "Sure, that was lovely. And it was great of you not to be uptight about it." Vic offered to make another round of drinks, trying to cover the awkward silence, but Dan pressed on.

"I'll bet you'd like to get your hands on her again, wouldn't you?"

No answer from Vic.

"Admit it," Dan continued. "Doesn't she have a great ass?" And with that Dan pulled you to him, spun you around, and before you knew it, had your skirt up, panties down, and your ass facing Vic.

"Honey, don't," you begged.

"You shouldn't be embarrassed," Dan said, anger tinting his voice. "I thought you liked fucking Vic."

You understood his plan now. He wanted to humiliate you and Vic in order to gain the upper hand. You tried to say something, but he was determined.

"You know what I'd like?" he asked to neither of you in particular. "I missed that other time. I'd like to watch the two of you making it."

Vic began to protest along with you. Exhibitionism wasn't your thing, and you were shocked to hear this from Dan.

"I'm serious." And he began to undress you in front of Vic. Suddenly you felt very shy and began to turn red. This egged Dan on even more.

"Look, she's blushing! Just like a virgin!" Vie could only stand and stare. He never took his eyes away. As your skirt and panties were removed, his attention was riveted to your blonde bush. Was that him breathing so heavily? And then Dan pulled off your sweater. Underneath you were bare. Your nipples had hardened and the area around them was very pink. You'd always been very proud of your breasts, but now you wanted to hide their fullness.

This wasn't wasted on Vic who had an enormous bulge in his pants.

Dan started to coax. "Listen, she told me you've got quite a weapon. That true?"

Vic, now very aroused, responded by pulling off his shirt. There was tight curly hair on his ebony chest. As he opened his pants, his Herculean black cock shot straight out. Dan was silent, but recovered as he pushed Vic towards you. Vic needed little guiding. You were staring at his marvelous instrument which had given you so much pleasure before. Just the memory made you lubricate. The two of you moved as if magnetized.

You knelt in front of him, his great cock hovering over you. You looked up at it and gently began licking, first underneath and then the tip which had a glistening drop at its opening. You licked it all over and fondled his balls as he sighed. Dan stood and stared as if watching a film. He began to touch himself almost unconsciously.

You kept licking Vic's cock and balls and then all at once took him in your mouth as far as he'd go. He started making love to your mouth. His eyes closed. No longer were you uneasy with your one-man audience. You just did whatever was natural.

After what seemed like a long time, Vic picked you up and laid you on the bed. He moved between your legs. Parting them wide, he placed his fingers at your opening and felt how wet and ready you were. He couldn't wait. He lifted you slightly and placed your legs on his shoulders as he entered. You gasped as that large, hard piston seemed to tear your apart — and feel beautiful too. There was no pain — only a kind of pounding of Vic in you, making you almost lose control of all senses.

Your bodies kept moving into all kinds of positions. Once you were sitting up on him, leaning your breasts so that the nipples kept flicking lightly against his dark chest. Dan moved closer now and you heard him undressing as he stood next to you. You became very conscious of the contrast your pale blondness made against Vic's charcoal flesh. It turned you on picturing it, and whatever else Dan's reaction was, it turned him on, too.

You were moving hard up and down on Vic, trying to force that giant member up the length of your body when something hard was against your back. Dan's erect penis brushed you. He didn't say a word but kept brushing against your back and buttocks all the while you moved up and down on Vic. Then Dan reached in front for your breasts and started to fondle them. He knew just how you liked the nipples to be squeezed and pulled, and this heightened your pleasure. He pushed you forward a bit, and was massaging your buttocks and asshole ever so slightly. He kept on and it was explosive.

Vic could see this new development and was getting more and more excited. With an unexpected movement, Dan inserted his cock into that tiny posterior opening. No! it would hurt, you pleaded, and it wasn't even possible . . . but Dan didn't care what you said. He continued pushing gently and then, he was in! It was unbelievable — Vic beneath you and Dan behind you. And it felt wilder and more wonderful than anything you'd ever experienced. You didn't dare change position as your three bodies meshed like some sort of mechanical contrivance going at an ever-quickening pace. You felt Vic moving in and out below and Dan pounding from behind. And suddenly Vic started to breath very heavily and to moan, "I'm going to come . . . As he did he touched off a chain reaction, for you joined him almost at once and a moment later Dan was shooting hot liquid into you as well.

You lay in each other's arms afterward and exchanged hugs and smiles. You saw that Dan had more than "evened" things out and jealousy was no longer a word that would pass between you three.

30

New Girl in Town

How long had it been since you'd gotten together with Sara? Could it really be three months? Ever since she called to say she was in town for a week and to ask if you could get together, you couldn't stop thinking about her. Funny how the two of you met in the first place. You, the young wife of an upcoming surgeon and she, the visiting girl friend of an artist. If he'd never shown his paintings at that gallery and if your husband hadn't reluctantly accepted the invitation, you probably never would have met.

How the two of you wound up in bed is almost as unlikely. Your husband was frankly turned on by her, and although the two of you had never participated in any group sex, circumstances just carried you in that direction. He had had a number of drinks when Sara's artist friend suggested that you all go to his place for a nightcap. It wasn't a big jump from a drink to some pot and then into bed. The biggest surprise came to you, however. You were all making love and exchanging mates, when the artist suggested the two girls kiss. Wow! You'd never done anything like it—and it hit you hard! At first you were reluctant, but soon you were eagerly kissing and stroking Sara, and she you.

But it was soon over. And it was a problem. What was going to happen to you? You had been turned on by a girl. Were you a lesbian? Were you sick? So many disconcerting questions without answers! And since your husband chose to completely eliminate the incident from his consciousness, there was no one to talk with about it.

Today, Sara called—it was the first time you'd had any contact with her since that unforgettable evening. You didn't even try to pretend you were busy. You knew you'd be seeing her, and although you were filled with guilt, you knew this was one appointment you were going to keep.

Sara named a hotel and a time, and as you dressed very carefully, you were afraid you'd forget—knowing you'd never forget. How does a woman dress to turn on another woman? A puzzling question. So you merely dressed as you would to please a man. It was that simple. You placed a bit of perfume on each breast and on the hair between your legs. Hmmm. Why was it perfume there turned you on?

Finally the hours fled and you were knocking at the hotel room door. Sara opened it and stood there for just a moment before taking your hand and then pulling you into her arms to embrace you. You felt shy and awkward. She sensed this and drew back. You sat down next to her on the bed, and she merely held your hands in hers and looked lovingly into your eyes. Then she kissed you, gently at first, until you—well, you felt comfortable with her. At that point she slowly undressed you, not speaking at all. You let her initiate the pace. First your shoes; then your lightweight summer dress. You didn't wear a bra, so there were only the bikini panties left, and soon these were off, too. Sara stood at the side of the bed admiring your body stretched out before her, then she undressed quickly and lay down next to you.

How can you describe that embrace? Your legs were entangled and your arms groped for one another. And the kisses. The kisses all over your face and your body, and you kissing her. It was like making love to yourself reflected in a sylvan pool.

Before long there was only one spirit—no leaders or followers. She made you lie on your back and began licking your body from your eyes to your neck to your breasts until you were panting and almost unable to contain yourself. You knew her kisses and licking would reach your very core and as you felt her tongue touch that most vulnerable part of you, your body arched and you nearly fainted. Within moments you convulsed in orgasm and she held you lovingly.

Then in automatic reciprocation you turned to pleasure her. Only she lay face down on the bed and you began your kissing from the soles of her feet upward to her calves and to the backs of her knees. You heard a low moan. You continued to kiss and lick upwards until you reached her buttocks. How lovely they were. Small but full, with not the least bit of hanging flesh. You lingered there kissing and licking and then gently spread the cheeks of Sara's lovely ass.

Now as if you'd done this a hundred times, you found yourself licking around her tiny anus which at first withdrew in reflex, but soon accepted the tip of your tongue. You licked it all around and then darted in and out while she sighed in delight. You moved slightly and let her raise her body to give you access to her delicious vagina.

You did all the things she did to you, licking slowly at first and only teasing her clitoris. Then you were more persistent and as you felt that button harden, you licked until you knew she was about to come. But she didn't want to let go just yet and so she gently moved your head away and rolled over.

"It's just about this time when we could use a man," she sighed.

You were hurt—wondering why she wasn't as delighted with you as you had been with her. As if reading your mind she said, "It's just that I really like to have a penis inside of me when I'm about to come." But since there was no man around, the problem seemed insurmountable.

"Wait a second. I've got an idea," Sara said and she moved to a bowl of fruit the hotel had thoughtfully provided.

"This will be our penis!" she said brightly as she brandished a medium-sized slightly unripened banana.

After examining it, you both decided it would be best to remove the peel, which didn't look very sanitary. Then Sara spread her legs wide apart. You lubricated her with your tongue to make easier entry for the surrogate penis. Its tip went in quite easily, but you were afraid it might break so you moved it very gingerly, only inserting a few inches. But when Sara kept moaning for more, you pushed the entire banana into her, with only the end tip showing. She pushed with her vaginal muscles and expelled it a bit, and you pushed it back into her. This began your rhythm. You moved so you could also caress the tip of her clitoris with your tongue, all the while thrusting the banana.

Her excitement was unbelievable. She moaned more than before and soon started to whisper, "I'm coming. I'm coming," until, with a beautiful rush, she climaxed. As she did, what was left of the banana was pushed out of her. You couldn't help yourself—you just put your tongue back into her and licked and licked until all the fruit was gone.

Soon after when you lay together on the bed, Sara told you that she would be moving back to town. You both smiled, knowing there would be many afternoons like the one you'd just spent.

31

Faithful Friends

JIM WAS AWAY on a fishing trip with some friends. It had been a slow, lazy evening. You'd watched some television and struggled over the crossword puzzle. You were about to step into the shower and get ready for bed when you heard the downstairs buzzer. You weren't expecting anyone, especially not Sue and Charlie, whose voices greeted you cheerfully over the intercom.

"We were in the neighborhood and since we knew Jim was out of town, we thought we'd say hello."

"Well, I was going to turn in . . ." you said lamely into the box on the wall. When there was no response, you felt bad about hurting their feelings. After all, they had only good intentions. So you filled the long pause, "Oh, okay, come on up."

You quickly ran through the apartment straightening up. You disliked people just dropping by, but you never could hurt anyone's feelings. Besides, you had been alone now for almost five days, and conversation other than the Friendly News Team's would be welcomed.

In they came, each giving you a kiss on the cheek before dropping onto the sofa. You offered drinks, which were accepted. As you were mixing them in the kitchen, you heard them whispering and giggling. You wondered what was so funny.

You usually weren't much of a drinker, but somehow one drink led to another, and you soon found yourself fixing a third round. Admittedly, you felt much more relaxed than you had in the past few days. You let your head rest on the back of the easy chair into which you had plopped.

Charlie got up to put on some records, and soon he and Sue were dancing. You watched as they moved, slowly and very close together. You couldn't take your eyes off of them, but they seemed oblivious of you. They were holding each other very tightly, dancing dreamily. When Charlie turned to you and asked you to join them, you blushed, wondering if he'd caught you staring at them. But he insisted until the three of you were standing in a tiny group, swaying to the music.

You hadn't realized how you missed Jim holding you. You started to tremble when Charlie put his arm around your waist. "Hey," he asked, "what's wrong?"

"Oh nothing," you replied. "I guess I just miss Jim, that's all."

"Well, maybe we can substitute," he said teasingly. He held you tightly so that you had little choice but to keep on dancing awkwardly in the center of the room.

The liquor was making you unsteady. You really wanted to sit down and said so. Charlie said no and somehow you couldn't resist him.

Before very long they changed positions, and you found yourself facing Charlie with Sue directly behind you. She pressed you against him and he held you tightly.

"Come on," you said uncomfortably, "what's going on?"

"Charlie thinks he knows what will be good for you," Sue explained. "Why don't you just relax?"

It dawned on you then that they had this set up beforehand. You pulled away and asked them to leave, saying you were tired and really wanted to go to bed now.

"We're not going anywhere," Charlie replied and he went to the door and fastened the chain lock. You couldn't understand any of this. As your anger began to rise, Sue took your hand

and led you out of the living room toward your bedroom. "Wait," you shouted. "Leave me alone and get out!"

No answer at all now, just Charlie grabbing your other hand and the two of them literally pulling you.

You were becoming a little frightened now. These were your old friends. Why were they acting this way?

Before you could think it through, Charlie was pushing you down on the bed. As you tried to rise, he slapped you across your face, hard, and you started to cry.

"Stop! Get out!" But of course, they didn't. Charlie took some rope from his pocket which he had obviously brought along just for this purpose. Sue then pushed you down on the bed again and tied your wrists to the headboard so that you couldn't move to defend yourself.

Sue followed Charlie's lead as they began to unbutton your robe. You had nothing on under it, and in a moment you were naked. Tears were running down your cheeks, but Charlie smiled and nodded to Sue. She got out of her dress quickly. He too undressed after tying your ankles to the bottom of the bed. You were now completely their victim.

Why wasn't Jim here? None of this could have been happening if he were.

Charlie reached down and grabbed at your large breasts. You closed your eyes, trying not to watch any of this. Sue was at your legs and started to caress the sensitive skin inside your thighs.

"We just want to keep you company while Jim is away," she purred. Their hands played until your body couldn't help but respond. It had been a long time since you'd had any sex and now, in the midst of this rape scene, you found yourself getting very wet and sticky.

She was at your pubic hair, brushing her fingertips against it gently. You found yourself arching, trying to reach her fingers. Sue saw this and deliberately started to tease you, withdrawing her fingers just as they were coming close. Oh how you wished you could just lie there numbly, but your body paid no attention to your mind.

Charlie was sucking at your breasts making your nipples very hard. You heard your breathing grow hoarse. You opened your eyes and saw Charlie hovering above you with a very large erection. It had been so long since you had any man other than Jim. You had been completely faithful to him for the three years you had been married. But the sight of Charlie's rigid penis was turning you on. You had been so lonely. . . .

Charlie moved his hand to where Sue's had been, and she replaced him at your breasts. As he touched you, you felt warm liquid gush from your body. You couldn't bear to look at him. He must be laughing at you. But all you could think about now was his penis, and you were hoping he would put it inside you. Instead, he kept playing with you, lightly encircling your clitoris until it was quite hard. You felt you were about to come.

Finally he withdrew his hand. You meekly tried to close your legs, your mind trying to regain control, but all it took was a gentle pressure from him for your legs to part and welcome him.

Sue was watching and was getting pretty worked up. She began playing with herself. But she wasn't going to interfere. This evening was apparently all for you.

You felt the tip of Charlie's penis at the entrance of your vagina. You couldn't help it. You let out a sigh as he pushed himself in a bit, torturing you, for all you wanted now was the full length of his hardness inside you. He took his time until you heard yourself begging, "Please, please, put it in."

"That's what I was waiting for," he said. Then he pushed it all the way in. All the air went out of you like a balloon which has just been pierced. Soon your moving pelvis was meeting his pummeling. "Faster," you whispered. He was close to you, pumping in and out very slowly and then faster in response to your demands.

It wasn't long before your climax was rising. You were a dam ready to burst free. Sue was right alongside the two of you playing with herself. As you came so did Charlie and a moment later Sue did, too. The three of you lay there drifting.

In a few moments they untied your hands and feet. You couldn't move as they dressed silently. They went to the door and were about to let themselves out, when you heard Charlie call back to you, "Anytime Jim is out of town, don't forget—you can count on us."

32

The $500 Assignment

JESUS, YOU WERE broke! Work was so difficult to find that when Fred called and told you he had a one-shot deal where you could make an easy $500, you agreed without even asking what you had to do.

Now you felt a bit foolish. You only had the address and the time to report and no idea of what to expect. You knew Fred was involved in many different kinds of deals—some involving the sex magazine he published—but you figured he wouldn't take advantage of your friendship.

Even before you rang the bell, you could hear voices. Your curiosity was piqued. Upon entering, you realized that this wasn't really an apartment—it was more like a photographer's studio. There were several cameras and solid white backdrops and about a half dozen men around the room, chatting, drinking and apparently having a good time.

"Are you the girl Fred sent?" someone asked.

"Yes," you replied, trying to figure it all out. He introduced himself briefly. "I'm the photographer. You can undress in that room over there, please."

You didn't comment but were a bit thrown.

You looked around again and saw that you were the only girl present. You got a little worried, but the thought of how far that $500 would go towards paying the pile of stacked-up bills stopped you from asking any questions that might jeopardize it.

You undressed. Finding no robe or costume to change into,

you shyly opened the door and tried to slip unnoticed into the larger room.

"Well, come on," the photographer said, and you hurried over. What am I getting myself into, you wondered?

"Look," you said quietly, "I don't really know what I'm supposed to do." Your voice trailed off.

"You're here to help us test rubbers," he replied. When you looked blankly at him, he explained, as if to a dumb child, "condoms, prophylactics, safes . . . And you have to keep the guys hard while I photograph them for a piece in Fred's magazine."

"I can't," you blurted out. "I didn't know.

The photographer looked annoyed and said, "Well, if you won't, get out, and we'll get someone else."

Again you thought about how much you needed that money and weighed it in your mind against your shocked sensibilities. What would your friends say if they found out? But you decided to stay.

The men started to undress and soon the photographer was the only one clothed. The first guy came up to you and simply pushed you down on your knees and said, "Suck it, baby, and get it up."

You were about to reply to his offhand attitude but were silenced by his limp penis being stuffed into your mouth. You didn't have much experience with oral sex, but here you were with some strange guy sticking himself into you. He held your head with both his hands so he could control his movements. After a while he was erect. Then he moved away and put on a rubber while the photographer set up the shot. He didn't look at you again.

The next guy came over and he too, simply positioned himself in front of you and instructed you to lick and suck him hard. This one also asked you to play with his balls. He had the same total lack of interest in you as the first guy. You realized quickly that all you were was a mouth—a machine to get them hard, so they didn't have to do it themselves. You felt angry and confused.

You decided to give the next guy on the line a little surprise. You looked up at him and smiled. He didn't expect this and was startled. You kept your eyes on him as you fondled his penis before slipping it into your mouth. You were going to give this guy an erection that he wouldn't soon forget.

As he started to move automatically, you tightened your mouth around him, but held your teeth away from his very sensitive skin. You nibbled the tip of his penis and licked it all over, keeping up a steady light motion. He got hard quickly. You began to caress his balls and you felt his body now under your control. He seemed to forget why he was there as he moved in your mouth as if it were a vagina before him.

As you kept teasing him with your tongue, you sensed his orgasm was approaching. He moved faster and started to groan. The sound drew all eyes to you.

You pulled your mouth back and used your tongue again, letting them all see you lick the shaft and the balls—gently, ever so gently. As they watched you were surprised at your feeling of complete self-confidence. You were on stage and you were enjoying it. You decided to give them a real show. You began playing with yourself with your free hand, but never letting up on the hard rod in your mouth. Each time he was about to come, you took your mouth away gently and slowed him down.

Finally, you knew he couldn't keep it up much longer. You sucked harder and harder, all the while playing with his balls and with yourself.

"I'm coming!" he shouted. You sucked until you tasted the salty liquid pour into your mouth, making you gag slightly, but only for a moment. After that it tasted good and you drank him dry.

When you saw the others eying you, you decided that you liked your newfound job. You'd let it be known that you would do the same for all of them — that is, if they would help a girl out a bit with her expenses. . . .

33

He Gives You Away

IT'S EARLY EVENING and you're lying in bed listening to soft music on the radio. You're finding it difficult to concentrate on the suburban housewife articles in the magazine you were reading. You feel very horny tonight. You're tempted to play with yourself, but your boyfriend Eddie is in the next room playing poker with some men. There's only the bedroom door separating you, and he may walk in at any time.

You're torn from your daydreams when the door is flung open. He's standing over you. You look up at him and without warning he rips the covers from you. You're totally nude.

He's looking at you strangely. He has a feather in his hand which he uses to tickle you very lightly between your legs. You part them and you can feel yourself lubricating. You are longing for him, but again you're aware that he has a strange look about him. Suddenly he reaches down, takes you by the hair, and lifts your head from the pillow. Roughly he pushes you down to the floor on all fours.

"What are you doing?" you ask. "Your friends are in the next room!"

"Shut up," he says and gives your hair a yank. He gets behind you, still holding you by the hair so you're unable to move easily. You expect him to put his cock in you, but instead you feel only his fingers playing tauntingly around the outside of your vagina. You begin to sob softly with fear and frustrated desire.

"Over here," he says as he forces you to crawl over to the

dressing-room mirror. You watch his reflection unzip his pants and his cock thrusts itself out.

Holding your head tightly so that you must look into the mirror, he mounts you and begins to fuck you. He plunges with great energy and in abrupt uneven movements. You begin to moan with pleasure, but you still can't turn your head.

After a few moments he stops. Sounding a bit disgusted, he says, "It doesn't look like I'm coming, does it? Well I'd better do something to turn me on. Come with me." With that, he zips up his pants although you can see the outline of his hardon through his trousers. Then, still not permitting you to raise your head, he force-walks you on all fours into the next room. There are six men sitting in comfortable chairs. "How do you like it?" he asks them. "Beautiful," somebody says.

"What an ass," another comments. "Can I touch that ass?"

"Help yourself," he says.

And so the man reaches over and begins to pat one of your buttocks. Then he pulls both cheeks apart, revealing your asshole. One of the men reaches over and forces the tip of his finger into it. You can hear the men talking, but you are unable to turn to look because Eddie is still holding your head straight ahead.

"Isn't she a nice pet?" Eddie asks. "Who wants to fuck her?"

For a moment no one says anything, but soon someone takes the challenge. "I'd love it, if you're serious."

"Be my guest," your boyfriend says, and he turns you around so your ass is facing the man who was speaking.

You can hear his pants drop and he lowers himself and begins to fuck you. You're angry and indignant, but, in spite of this, you're very excited. Your eyes close as you slip into a state of just feeling. You feel yourself coming, but before you can, your head is yanked back by the hair.

"Suck this!" someone says and you are forced onto the cock

of one of the seated men. Others now reach over and begin playing with your breasts and ass as a free-for-all ensues.

They're pulling your nipples very roughly, getting you hotter and hotter while hurting you at the same time. You're sucking this stranger's cock as hard as you can while another is fucking you from behind. You are responding like a machine—taking anyone or anything that is presented to you. You can't even look to see whose hands are upon you.

The man behind you makes a final violent thrust and his semen shoots into you. He withdraws, but before you can catch your breath, another one is in you.

One after the other they fuck you, and as each new one sticks his cock in you, Eddie pulls your head over so that you have to suck someone as well. Soon you know that you're sucking some of the limp penises, the ones who've already been in you, and you can taste yourself. You like the taste, and it turns you on even more.

At last everyone has come in you at least once, and you have collapsed on the floor. Now Eddie stands behind you and lifts you up by the legs so that you're practically standing on your head. He begins to lick at your cunt. As the blood rushes to your head, you feel on the verge of blacking out. But it's a beautiful, joyful, unconsciousness, and suddenly you come and come and come and come. You're completely an animal. You hardly recognize the grunts and sounds issuing from you.

When it's over, he pushes you to all fours again and says, "I'm going to put her back in the cage now, fellows. I'll be with you in a minute."

You think he's joking, but he walks you into the bedroom that way and orders, "Wait here till I come back." You stay on your hands and knees for an hour before he finally returns. He lifts you up just as if you were a dog, tosses you onto the mattress, and fucks you beautifully. When he has finished you fall asleep in each other's arms.

34

The Caged Man

IT WAS VERY dark. All the audience could see was a dark mass up there on the stage. But as the spotlight came up, the mass began to take a more discernible shape. It was a cage in the center of the bare stage. In it was a very large, muscular black man with his hands shackled at the wrists and joined with a length of chain which barely gave him any freedom to move his hands. His feet were similarly restrained. He peered out at the audience, but the spotlight blinded him. It was clear that he was frightened. He tried to hide himself, but that was impossible.

A few moments passed when four young girls, none of whom could have been older than sixteen or seventeen, walked onto the stage. Each had been chosen for her voluptuous body. Their breasts were held in the tiniest bras, made of the sheerest fabric, revealing more than they covered. One slight breeze would have probably disintegrated them. The girls all had wide hips and firm, round buttocks. Their panties were hardly more than G-strings. They wore high black boots.

They walked from the corners of the stage towards the cage. An inhuman moan was heard from the man; he seemed to be frantic.

An amplified voice suddenly filled the room, making the audience jump.

"This man has been caged for eight months. In all that time he has not seen a woman. Guards stationed round the clock have kept him from even touching himself."

The man stared at the girls — as if they were some strange creatures. His glance kept darting from one to another. And they moved closer and closer to the cage.

One girl took a large key from around her waist and unlocked the door. At first the man cowered in the corner, obviously confused and afraid. He hadn't been out of this cage for so long. What was expected of him? She reached in and led him by the hand to the center of the stage. The other girls joined her. A large board was brought forward and before he could react, they had fastened his hand and leg shackles to it. He could not move.

One by one each girl removed the little bit of clothing she wore. And each one paraded in front of the man as she slowly stripped. One was blonde. As she disrobed, he seemed to be devouring her with his eyes. Her hair was very long, reaching to her waist. As she undressed he could see that her pubic hair was also blonde. She stroked it and teasingly offered it up to him. Instantly his penis was hard. The girl let her blonde bush brush lightly against his large, black cock. He would have climaxed had she not suddenly slapped his penis very hard so that he lost his erection.

As quickly as she moved away, the brunette was upon him. She had already disrobed and now turned her back to him so that her ass touched the tip of his cock. When she felt a drop of hot liquid about to shoot forth, she turned away and quickly squeezed him to make him lose his erection again.

The redhead was next. She almost pushed away the other girl in her eagerness. She had the largest breasts of the group and could lift them up and suck her own nipples. She performed as she knelt at his feet, placing herself right between his legs. As she looked up at him provocatively, she watched his penis grow hard again. It seemed to grow larger with each new erection, and his face showed true physical pain. His body strained forward, trying to reach the girl, but he could not. He began to sob.

The last girl stepped forward. She had short, brown hair and was very slender. She removed every article of flimsy clothing except her high boots. As she strutted before him, she revealed a riding crop which she kept slapping into her hand. As she passed him, she lightly struck him, first across the chest, then the thighs, and finally on the tip of his penis. He cried out in pain once more as she continued to walk back and forth.

Now the others joined her. They all seemed to work on him at once. One of them began kissing him hard on the mouth and stuck her tongue deep into him. But each time he would try to respond, they stopped him. Another girl was stroking his chest and licking at his nipples while another fondled his balls. And the last began to lick at his cock. They were in complete control of him. Whenever they saw he was about to explode in orgasm, they drew away and prevented him. He was crying and moaning like an animal rather than a human. He pleaded for release but they ignored him.

Finally the audience, responding to the man's desperation, seemed to be unable to take any more frustration. They shouted to let him come, let him come!

It was then that a fifth girl appeared. She somehow incorporated all of the fantastic qualities of each of the others. She was beautiful, with huge, high breasts and large nipples which stood out hard. Her legs were long and slender. Her hair was black and luxuriant. She walked up to him. He seemed about to lose consciousness. As she approached, he came to life once more. Now he was truly an animal. As she neared, they unlocked him. He leaped at her with a savage growl.

Never had the audience seen such a huge cock. Freed of his shackles they saw the man he really was. In spite of his imprisonment, he was astonishingly muscular. He stood tall for the first time and he was large and handsome. His black-ness was in shocking contrast to the white skin of the last girl.

His power matched hers and he pounced upon her. He threw her to the floor of the stage and thrust himself into her with such violence it seemed he would go right through her. She gasped in pain at first and then she clasped her legs tightly around his waist as he started to move with no stopping. He was a machine. And yet he had perfect control. He groped for her breasts and fed at them hungrily with his mouth. They were united—moving with a single will.

When he started to come, it was as if a dam was let loose. Eight months of abstinence was ended. He groaned loudly and wouldn't stop coming as his pumping never let up.

Afterwards he collapsed on the stage. He didn't move for a long time. But as he began to, he felt his wrists and ankles being chained once again and he was carried back into the cage. As the curtain closed, all the audience could hear was the soft sound of sobbing.

35

The Third Way

THE EVENTS OF that evening were pretty hazy. You were very drunk but were sober enough to realize that Jerry had deliberately egged you into drinking as much as you had. He was always coming down hard on you for being uptight and having all sorts of inhibitions. It was a constant source of argument between you. He kept telling you how "different" you were in bed after a few drinks, but you refused to believe it.

In the back of your mind you wondered if Jerry wasn't cooking up something by getting you high. But you'd drunk too much to follow the thought through. You realized foggily that one minute he was putting bottles away and now suddenly you were in his bedroom without being sure whether you walked in yourself or he carried you in in his arms.

He was helping you undress. Boy! You were really smashed! But you were feeling good, too, and kittenish. As he took your clothing off, you grabbed playfully at his crotch. You kept tickling him and rubbing his hairy stomach as he removed your things. It always turned him on to undress you. Now he had to do the job without any help from you, you were such a rag doll.

Finally, when you were nude, Jerry began to run his hands over your body. You knew what would come next—first your face and neck and then your shoulders. Shoulders were a big thing—your secret erogenous zone—and Jerry kissed them lightly as the goosebumps rose all over you. Next your breasts—he had remarked when you first got together about the largeness of your nipples which stood out so hard and firm when excited. Now he was pulling at them with his lips, taking care not to hurt, just hard enough to feel good.

He went down your body pausing briefly at your navel, your thighs, and calves and working back up to your crotch. It was odd that as dark as your hair was on your head, your bush was very scant, and the lips of your vagina were clearly visible. He kissed you on your appendix scar. You recalled vaguely how Jerry had refused to allow you to think of it as ugly. "It's part of you," he always said, "so it's lovely and interesting and just as beautiful as the rest of you." Tonight he was in a hurry to have you lie on your stomach. You dreamily turned and he stroked your back and buttocks all the way down to your heels. You felt him working upwards and playing around your ass again and you wondered why. Then he spread your legs wider and began to concentrate on your anus. You recoiled. You didn't want that! You even said it out loud. But Jerry was persistent.

"Don't worry, honey, it won't hurt."

"Please don't, Jerry," you begged. "It's . . . dirty. I don't like it."

But Jerry continued no matter how you tried to dissuade him. He sat on your legs holding you firmly as he positioned himself right below your buttocks so you couldn't move away.

"I've always wanted to get in there. . . ." You felt disgusted—how could anyone want to touch you . . . there!

But the more you squirmed, the more he held you. Soon you felt his finger circling your tiny asshole and poking in a little bit.

"Ouch!" you cried out. It was more uncomfortable than painful. He removed his finger, wet it, and then started again. This time he played for a long time around the rim and you felt oddly expectant. It was tantalizing. When he next inserted his finger, it didn't hurt as much as the first time. He pushed it in further and your sphincter muscle, which had tightened against this intrusion, began to relax. In a little while you felt his finger go all the way in with no resistance from you.

Soon he inserted two fingers and probed steadily. At this point he shifted his weight, and you felt his hard cock up against your ass. It was satiny as he put it between your buttocks and rubbed it there, too. You were really getting heated up.

He moved then and you expected to feel him inside your cunt. Instead, he was pushing against your anus—as he had done with his fingers.

"It's too big, you'll tear me apart—"

DON'T!

But there was no stopping Jerry now, He reached for a jar of cold cream from the night table and greased up his cock. He had such a large one, you could picture it tearing you open.

He put the head against your asshole and pushed a bit. As it entered you felt nothing but pain. All the muscles in your body tensed and tried to expel him. But he kept going. He pushed it in further and you groaned—not with pleasure, but in real agony.

"Relax," he kept saying, but all you could think of was how it was hurting you.

He continued to push the rest of his cock in until your body adjusted to it. Once again you felt yourself relax. As he felt less resistance, he pushed further. All at once, with one great thrust he was in up to the hilt. You gasped as you felt his cock being swallowed up into your ass. Then a strange thing happened. You began moving back and forth, no longer fighting it, but helping him. You were having the most incredible feelings that ranged between pain and delight. It was awful—and wonderful all at once. You felt yourself break out into a cold sweat, and you felt Jerry pushing and grunting and sweating, too.

You moved faster to meet his thrusts while he moved one hand around to massage your clit. It quickly hardened. He kept up his circular massage while moving in and out of your tight ass. Each time he withdrew, you felt the walls close up, and when he entered, they pushed open again. It was tighter than your cunt, and felt more slippery. You were getting very excited and strange sounds were coming from you.

As you came closer and closer to orgasm, Jerry kept up his clit massaging and the steady tempo with his cock. When you came, it was the most incredible orgasm you could remember. Almost immediately he came in your ass and slumped on top of you.

You both were exhausted afterward. Why had you waited so long to open the door to this new and intriguing sensation?

36

Uncle Arthur

EVERYONE ELSE HAS said goodnight. You've lingered a few extra seconds watching Angela, the pert young Nubian maid, clear away the dinner dishes. But now you, too, blow a kiss to your uncle and go up to your room to prepare for bed.

You take your usual long, leisurely bath, but tonight you add a few drops of perfumed oil to the hot water. Because tonight is different. Tonight, if you can summon up the courage, you're going to give your Uncle Arthur the surprise of his life.

For years you've had a schoolgirl crush on your mother's younger brother. Everytime he has visited the family for a few days, you've watched him furtively, passionately fantasizing about his strong arms, his warm passionate lips, the glow in his eyes. His dark stylishly long hair, his tall trim body are all so appealing to you. And yet he doesn't pay much attention to you. He thinks of you only as his "kid niece."

Tonight he's going to pay attention!

You made this decision a couple of days ago on your sixteenth birthday. Age is not going to make any difference. Nor is the kinship. So you soak in the bath longer than usual, feeling delicious and yet trembling with anxiety. When you finally stand up from the now-tepid water, you carefully towel-dry your firm young body and scrutinize yourself carefully in the mirror on the bathroom door. Looking at yourself turns you on. Your raven hair, which falls straight to below your shoulders, is matched in color by the full curly bush between your legs. Even as you rub your hand lightly over the black triangle, it glistens with water droplets from the bath. Tonight, you sigh softly, you'll make your move.

Later, you wait in your room until you're sure everyone has gone to sleep. Eventually the noises in the house subside and everything is very quiet. To be certain, you give yourself another ten minutes, while you imagine how it's going to be. You have to change your thoughts, for you're getting so excited you can almost feel the wetness trickling from between your legs.

At last the time has come. You urge yourself forward to keep from losing your nerve. It's now or never.

You tiptoe to Uncle Arthur's room and press your ear against the door. Hearing nothing, you very gently turn the handle and slip inside. Light from the moon falls on his bed, and he's apparently asleep, only a light sheet covering him. He's moved around so that one of his firm buttocks is exposed. You want to reach down and kiss it. At the same time you're fighting the urge to run out of the room. What if he gets angry? What if he shouts? What if—?

As if in answer to your fears and questions, your uncle opens his eyes. As he focuses on you, he gasps, "Hey, kid, what are you doing here?"

"I—I—couldn't sleep," you reply lamely. "Can I sit on the bed and talk to you?"

"Well. . . I guess . . .," he answers.

So you sit down and begin to talk. What you're saying is so inane it makes you both smile, but before either of you can comment on the quality of the conversation, your hand has dropped to his thigh. You act as if you're totally unaware of doing it, but slowly you move your fingers up on the sheet until you're just inches away from his penis. You keep talking about the weather and the moon and the local drought. Then you turn slightly so that your hand covers those couple of inches and rests on his penis. You feel as if you have a live snake beneath you as it suddenly hardens.

"Hey!" your uncle sputters. "Hey!" But before he can say another "hey," you pull aside the sheet and bury your head on top of his penis. Your tongue caresses its tip. "Christ!" is all he can say now. You take the first four inches into your mouth and lovingly move on them, sucking his penis as if it were a Popsicle. You reach down to slowly tickle and caress his balls. He moans again, and then he grabs one of your large breasts and pulls at its nipple ever so beautifully.

You are so involved in what you're doing that neither of you hears the door open. You both are aware of it simultaneously. But the moment of panic is replaced by surprise — it's Angela, the maid.

"What are you doing here Angela?"

She looks directly into your uncle's eyes. "Well, Miss, I'm doing what I always do, but it seems as though you've gotten here first. I suppose there's no room for me." Your uncle looks at you for just a second and then says, "Don't be silly, Angela, come over and join the party."

As quickly as that she leaps onto the bed, pulling off her nightgown, and begins sucking at the cock that has just been in your mouth. You have a feeling of girlish competitiveness and reach to push her aside. But as you do, your hand brushes her black breast. It feels so good that you find yourself caressing it. Slowly her head turns and the penis falls out of her mouth. She looks up at you with longing. You bend down and kiss her passionately on the lips again and again. It's obvious that you don't want to part, but then your uncle takes charge. He plays with both of you before turning you onto your back. He begins to fuck you and then Angela who's lying at your side. As he alternates fucking one and then the other, you and Angela kiss and play with each other's breasts.

At long last Uncle Arthur comes. He's standing up and using his penis as if it were a hose, squirting the cum on both of you. You love it.

He sighs a little as the last drops splash down. Angela and you reach over and pull him to the bed and the three of you, arms entwined, kiss each other. You smile to yourself thinking about how just a little courage, just a little daring, has resulted in this marvelous experience that you know you'll never, never forget.

37

Soft Cock

BEN AND YOU had been dating for a month. You really liked him, despite his slight prudishness. It pleased you to know he was a gentleman, but, after all, neither of you were teenagers who needed to play games about sex.

You were a little worried that he had done no more than hold your hand and give you a goodnight kiss. When you broached the subject, he had a logical reason for taking it slow; he didn't really like to get physically involved until he felt he knew a girl well. (This actually flattered you and was a refreshing change from the usual rush act most men were compelled to come on with.)

So you had decided to wait and see how things developed naturally. But now you were at the point where you were left very horny after the ten-minute necking session that ended each date.

Tonight, you decided, would be different. You had invited him to your apartment, making sure your roommate would be out. The dinner was delicious but light. The wine was right; the music and lights soft. Ben seemed to relax more and more as the evening wore on, and you tried to be very seductive without coming on too strong.

Finally, you were lying in his arms on the rug in front of your fireplace, listening to the music and returning his kisses. You made an obvious show of your excitement as he continued to kiss you, very expertly. You took his hand and moved it to your breast, and after a moment's pause, he began to fondle it.

At first he was very gentle, but as you responded, he became more daring, kneading and brushing over your nipple until you were very excited.

After a long time he opened a few buttons of your blouse and put his mouth where his hands had been. He sucked at each nipple, taking your small, firm breasts in his mouth.

You moved so your body was pressing up against his, but he didn't take the cue. Instead, he started to work down your body very slowly. He kissed you all over. His lips glided over your rib cage and down to your navel where he permitted his tongue to explore. He continued downward, pausing long enough to kiss and lightly lick your protruding hipbones. You helped him to remove the rest of your clothing. You had expected him to undress, too, but when he didn't, you said nothing, thinking he might be worried about shocking you.

He did, however, continue to arouse you. He teased your hairy triangle by kissing and stroking all around, but saving it for last. Then he turned you over and let his fingertips play over your buttocks.

"You have a beautiful ass," he whispered, and he began to massage it.

You felt his tongue play around your asshole gently licking at it until it relaxed and opened to his urging. He inserted the tip of his tongue and moved it in and out like a tiny penis. You had never experienced this before and liked it very much.

After a while he turned you onto your back and started to kiss your bush again. You were breathing quite audibly now and begged him to stop teasing you.

"I can't stand it. Please put it in."

But he paid no attention. Instead he applied his tongue expertly to your clitoris and entire vaginal area. He licked and slurped and had you incredibly turned on. And then you begged again, "Please, I want you inside of me."

For some reason he stopped doing everything and sat

without moving. When you asked him what was wrong, he didn't seem able to look at you.

"Don't you like me?" you asked, confused.

"Of course, I like you—very much," he replied, still not looking at you. "It's just that. . ."

"Please tell me," you begged.

"Well, I've never been able to really have sex with a girl because I can't stay hard." This was a very painful admission.

You were silent for a couple of seconds and then said, "Let me see if I can't get you to relax enough to try—just try."

For the first time since he started this "confession," he looked at you directly and nodded agreement.

Now it was your turn. He took your place on the rug and you started kissing him. When he reached up to touch you, you gently discouraged him until he knew that this was going to be all for him.

You kissed him tenderly as you undressed him. You kissed his nipples as he had done yours, and it pleased you to see them get very erect. He just closed his eyes as you went on. There was no rush, and eventually you could see his body relax.

When you removed his pants he became self-conscious but your reassuring stroking put him at ease once more. As you massaged him all over, purposely avoiding his penis, you watched his face soften.

You told him to turn over as you had done before. You traced the line of his buttocks with your fingertips, ending your journey at his anus. You used your tongue, too. Although he tightened at first, you began to hear his murmurs of passion.

When he turned on his back, you saw that his penis was getting hard. You started to stroke him, beginning with his toes and working upward, still not touching his penis or testicles. You moved gingerly across his chest, and your tongue joined your hands in this exploration. You were arousing yourself as much as you hoped you were turning him on.

Then, very, very gently you let the tips of your fingers brush along his penis. Back and forth, back and forth, feather touches until he was totally at ease. At that point you leaned over and licked him lightly and then held his balls firmly, but gently, in one hand.

When he accepted this, you put your mouth over his penis and sucked ever so lightly. He let himself go completely now. You felt him growing in your mouth and getting very hard. He knew it and seemed to go along totally now. You sucked him slowly until you felt he was very firm.

"Would you like to come inside me?" you whispered, still stroking him gently.

"Yes ..he breathed, almost inaudibly.

So you continued. But you took your time, as you had all along. First you sat on top of him, near his penis, but did not insert it. You kept massaging it with your hand. Then you raised yourself up and let the tip of him just touch the outside of your vagina. God! You felt like ramming it into you, but you didn't dare. Instead, you lowered yourself onto him and sat there. He seemed to be waiting for your next move, but his body took over for him and he started slowly thrusting.

You now returned *his* movements as he grew harder and firmer with each thrust. His hands reached out for your breasts, and his motions became automatic. He moved in and out and the look of sheer delight on his face was enough to get you excited along with him.

As he moved faster and faster, you knew he would soon be coming. You aided him by matching his rhythm precisely. All at once he groaned. His body jerked violently as he came into you. His semen poured out endlessly, as if for all the times he had been unsuccessful. When his orgasm subsided, he lay back smiling.

You snuggled in his arms and knew that you had initiated him into a very long and loving relationship.

38

Adventure Uptown or Black Is Beautiful

You started the evening with a few cocktails, and you were feeling a little high. You had deliberately wandered into this strange, rough neighborhood seeking some kicks. Why you were there was a long story.

For as long as you were aware of sex, you had always had one recurrent fantasy: to enter into a place where no one knew you and to do brazen things you'd never dare to do in your "real life." It was a sort of Jekyll and Hyde fantasy, for in reality you were very shy and inhibited—a far cry from the domineering woman of your daydream. For a long time you didn't really believe you'd ever do it, but the fantasy had become more and more real and compelling. Lately it had become almost an obsession. Early this evening you decided to act it out so that it would stop plaguing your imagination all the time. In a few brave minutes you had choreographed the whole thing—and this was your bravest hour. If nothing else, just the fact that you had courage enough to try something this daring pleased you.

Now you were right in the midst of the action. You had dressed provocatively in a very tight, sexy dress with the highest-heeled shoes you owned. You had doused yourself with lots of perfume that had a particularly tantalizing name. None of it was wasted as you walked into the bar.

When you entered, most of the conversational murmur stopped and eyes turned in your direction. The hostility almost drowned you. You were an intruder in this world. But it never occurred to you to do an about face and leave. You just stuck your chin out arrogantly, walked over to the bar, and asked if they served Amaretto.

As the bartender poured, you felt eyes appraising your body. You were confident that you were being given high grades. You were quite tall and very slender. As slim as you were, though, your ass jutted out at a fetching angle and now was pressed hard against the tight fabric of your satin dress. Your legs were great; long and firm, curving just right, down to your slim ankles. None of it was missed by the crowd. You turned as you sipped your drink, letting them have the front view—small firm breasts which didn't need a bra to hold them high, a tiny waist, and a very attractive face with large blue eyes. Your hair was long and brown and practically reached your waist. You felt the few women in the place staring at you with hostility, but the men watched lustfully.

The crowd seemed to be waiting for a signal to resume their activity when suddenly one man stepped forward.

"What you want here?" he asked. "You no hooker. You belong downtown."

"I belong where I decide to go," you countered.

"Well," he asked, "you think you belong here?"

"Of course I came to sample some black cock!"

Someone at the end of the bar uttered a nervous laugh and someone else echoed it. You began to feel a little dizzy over your own brazenness. Perhaps your situation was more dangerous than you were aware of. . . .

"How about me?" the man asked with a leer, breaking the tension.

"You'll have to let *me* decide after I take a look."

Without hesitation—before the entire bar—he unzipped his fly and held out his enormous cock, which was already on its way to stiffness.

You examined it coolly and said, "Come closer."

He took a step forward.

"Not bad," you said. "Get it *really* hard."

"How about you doing that?" he suggested.

"I'll give the orders," you said firmly. When there was no response, you told the rest of the people to make a circle around one of the tables. They got right into it, and before long a stage was set.

"I'll undress you," you said, and you led him to the center of the circle. First you removed his shirt revealing his muscular chest. You stroked him, his arms, his back, his chest—not caressingly, but appraisingly. He stood flattered but confused. It was obvious that he usually made the demands.

You finished undoing his pants and took them off. Soon he was totally nude—except for his undershirt. His huge cock was standing up at five past six.

"Undress me," you demanded, "but touch only the clothes."

He followed your instructions precisely. In short order you were standing there naked except for your black stockings, black lace garter belt, and high, high heels.

As you lay down on the table, you ordered, "Move your ass over here and lick my nipples!" He was more than eager to please and took each nipple, and then each breast, into his mouth which seemed to swallow you up. He did his job well for soon you felt your cunt lubricate, and your body was getting increasingly sensitive to his touch.

"Now go down on me and start jerking yourself off."

He quickly got between your legs and lapped away until you were at the verge of coming. At the same time he pulled mercilessly at his rod.

"Stop!" you demanded and he immediately withdrew his tongue.

"Now shove that black cock into me!"

His firm stick was waving slightly over you as you opened

your legs wide. He first put the head in, very gently as if he didn't want to hurt you—your slit seemed so small. But that wasn't what you wanted.

"All of it—and fast," you yelled.

With one movement, he pushed his entire length into you. It was thick. You felt as if it would go straight through you. This was what you had fantasized about over and over, and now it was a delicious reality.

"Fuck me!" you pleaded. There was no holding him back now. His cock was like a piston as it moved around in you. You raised your legs and wrapped them around his waist, virtually becoming part of his body. The hands of some of the spectators were caressing your ass but you didn't object. You were on display and you loved it.

You heard his breathing getting louder, but you didn't want him to come—not just yet, not until you did—so you told him firmly to slow down.

Then you closed your eyes and concentrated . . . as if standing outside of yourself, you could see what the crowd saw: two total strangers fucking for this audience.

You loved the fucking, but you didn't ever reach orgasm that way. So as he screwed you, you began rhythmically fingering your clitoris as only *you* knew how to do. You couldn't care less if he might be put off. But as you opened your eyes a bit you saw he was fascinated by this. That excited you even more and as he moved his cock in and out of you, your fingers quickened and you knew it would be only moments before you came.

He continued to thrust, and you felt yourself getting closer and closer until you were coming and your rhythm quickened.

"Now!" you said loudly and he immediately moved faster. This time he grunted and groaned as he moved and you felt him shoot into you. Your body shook beneath him as wave after wave of your orgasm washed over you.

Then he lay still atop you and you felt other hands pulling at your tits. After a while he pulled out. You stared in admiration at his limp cock as he sank into a nearby stool and reached for his pants.

As he sat there you stood up and looked around. You put on your dress swiftly, adjusted your hair and makeup. With a slight smile in his direction, and then at the others, you walked directly to the door, and out to the street, never turning back for a second glance.

Since *To Turn You On* was written by a woman for women, it was not designed to please males. A few did have a chance to read the original script. If they objected to anything, invariably it was to the story you've just shared. They were offended. They were angered. They were indignant. "No woman could have such a fantasy," was their theme. If only for that reason, I marked it a "must include." Men have been dictating women's fantasies far too long!

39

Pay for Play

THE PLAN WAS for you to get into the city sometime in the afternoon and meet Paul in the lobby of the Hilton Hotel. You'd catch a film and have dinner before returning home on the 10:04 upstate. Of course the one thing you hadn't figured on was the train getting you there an hour and a half early. You might have killed time shopping, but you just couldn't make another trip to the stores when you were trying to economize. Luckily you had brought a paperback along, and you decided to just sit and wait in the hotel's lobby.

It was crowded with many check-ins and check-outs as well as friends meeting friends. This certainly seemed to be the central rendezvous spot in town. You couldn't help feeling that the tall blond guy hear the newsstand was trying to get your attention. He kept walking back and forth in front of you every few minutes. Although you tried to ignore him by focusing on your book, it became exasperating.

Finally he caught your eye. He seemed to be summoning up some courage as he walked towards you. Not bad looking, you thought. If you were single, you might even go for someone like him. You were halfway into your next thought when he spoke, "Do you come here often?" he asked.

"To a hotel lobby?" you replied. You thought his was a pretty silly question.

"Well, I was wondering if you were interested in making some extra money. . . ." His voice trailed off as he smiled.

In a flash you understood. He thought you were a hooker sitting there waiting to pick someone up.

"You have some nerve," you said, insulted.

"Take it easy," he said, "I only thought you were here . . . well professionally. You're really great looking, you know." He tried to smooth it over. "How about making an exception . . .?" he couldn't resist making another pitch.

"What do you think I am?" You tried to hold back your anger.

"Two hundred bucks is nothing to sneeze at," was all he said.

The whole scene was absurd. But when he said "two hundred bucks," somehow it seemed more ridiculous to you that a woman could spend a half hour with a guy and wind up richer for doing what she might very well enjoy doing anyway.

It had a crazy attraction. Who would know? Paul wasn't due to meet you for nearly an hour. You felt your heart racing. As the blond turned to leave, you blurted out, "I think I'll take you up on that offer." Was that actually your voice you heard? Before you could change your mind, he drew close, "I'm in room 603. I'll go up and you follow in a few minutes."

In those few minutes you decided to leave and changed your mind fourteen times. Were you crazy? Still, the idea was very titillating. You found yourself walking towards the elevator, entering, and pushing "six" almost like a robot.

You knocked lightly on the door which opened immediately.

He had his jacket off and offered you a drink, which you refused. Since you didn't know what to expect, you decided to leave it up to him.

He took off your jacket before leading you to the bed. You both sat down side by side and he did that number they do in the movies, taking your chin in one hand and tipping it up as he kissed you, lightly.

Zap! Electricity charged through you. Another kiss, heavier this time and he was pushing you back onto the bed. He kissed you all over your face and down your throat and you shivered with lovely feelings.

He then led your hand to his pants for you to unzip him. This was done deftly and reaching your hand inside, you managed to get beneath his jockey shorts to his two silky balls. He sighed with enjoyment. You felt for his penis which still lay limp. It stirred at your touch, and you played with it for a moment.

You parted briefly for him to remove his clothing and you followed, peeling off your slacks and sweater. You were standing in bra, panties, and shoes (silently congratulating yourself for dieting away those nine pounds) when he reached for you.

"I want to take the rest off," he said.

He unhooked your bra, allowing your breasts to fall free. The nipples were pink and sticking out. He kissed them lightly before removing your panties. He seemed surprised to see you were a natural redhead, and your fair bush was soon smothered by his kisses.

He was fairly good looking. You judged him to be about thirty-six. Although he was quite thin, he had the lean muscular look of an athlete. You had never seen a blond guy undressed, and it amused you to see his pubic hair nearly as fair as that on his head.

He drew you close to him, running his hands over your back and down to your jutting buttocks. He held them tightly, almost hurting you. He ground his body against you until he started to get quite firm. You parted again and he lay down on the bed.

"Go down on me," he said simply.

You hesitated, all of a sudden trying to remember who you were and wondering what you had gotten into.

"I said go down on me!" he ordered this time, taking your head and pushing it down to his body. He was uncircumcised, and his foreskin still covered part of the glans in its semierectness. You gingerly put your mouth over it. It had a pleasant, smooth feeling as you ran your tongue over it. He smelled good too, having the memory of talcum powder about him.

You took to your task quite eagerly and he got even harder in your mouth. It fit well and soon filled that opening completely. As you moved your head along the length of his penis, you stroked his balls. He sighed again. He grabbed your head by the hair.

"Lick my balls," he commanded. After some time, he pulled your head away. "That was good," he sighed. "Now lie on your back." You followed instructions. He positioned himself, missionary style, between your spread legs.

He had wasted no time playing with you, but since the whole scene had turned you on, you were well lubricated. He had no trouble entering.

As you felt him strike against your cervix, you had a sensation of total pleasure. This stranger who didn't care who you were and was merely using your body was really turning you on!

As he continued his movements, you started to play with yourself. He noticed and it seemed to excite him. It wasn't long before your clitoris was almost as hard as he was! You kept rubbing as he thrust into you and as you did, his cock pushed against your fingers. You got into a steady rhythm, which engulfed you.

"Come now," he whispered. "Come on, come on, come . . ."

His words got you even more excited, and you felt yourself coming as he continued entreating.

You felt the pulsations go on and on as he now pumped in and out of you faster and faster. Within moments he groaned, went rigid for an instant, and you felt his body shake as he poured into you. He collapsed on top of you.

A few moments later, as you dressed and fixed your makeup, he approached silently.

"Here," he said, thrusting something towards you. It actually took you a minute to realize it was money! You'd almost forgotten how this all started. "It was real good," he added. "You earned your money." You were amazed to note that all this had taken exactly forty minutes. And now you sat in the lobby again waiting for Paul, who would never in his wildest dreams imagine how you had spent part of this afternoon. You wondered if you might make plans to meet again in the city soon . . . maybe even next week.

Afterword

I **HOPE YOU'VE FOUND** personal pleasure in some of my fantasies. I hope too that they have stimulated your imagination so that you'll create a new assortment of your own private fantasies and thus expand the world of your own satisfaction.

The purpose of this book was to turn you on. If I have succeeded, even in part, then this isn't the end.

For you, it can be a whole new beginning!

.